FROM CRAZY TO CALM

Natural Ways To Boost Your Mental Health

Top Leaders Share
Their Expertise for Living a Calm,
Peace-Filled Life.

Shelly Jo Spinden Wahlstrom

And Other Leading Experts

FROM CRAZY TO CALM

Natural Ways To Boost Your Mental Health

Shelly Jo Spinden Wahlstrom

And Other Leading Experts

First Printing: June 2023

ISBN: 978-1-7362176-6-5

Shelly Jo Spinden Wahlstrom

Shelly Jo Hypno Aminos, LLC

PO Box 593

Roy, UT 84067

Hypnoaminos.com

shellyjo@hypnoaminos.com

Shelly Jo Spinden Wahlstrom is available to speak at your business or conference events on various topics. Email shellyjo@hypnoaminos.com for booking information.

Table of Contents

Why Read This Book?

"From Crazy to Calm: Natural Ways to Boost Your Mental Health" is a book that can help you find answers to feel better when you're feeling stressed, anxious, or down.

Through several top experts, you'll receive tips and ideas that you can use in your everyday life to improve your mental health and feel calmer and happier.

The goal of this book is to open your eyes to alternative tools to bring optimal health. Traditional options have their place, and so do alternative options. It allows you to see that there are many different alternatives to traditional medicine.") Yet, until you know the options, you may not know you have choices.

Reading this book may help you to understand your own mental health better and you'll learn to take care of yourself in a way that feels good and right for you. This book also shares stories of other people who have struggled with their own health and found ways to feel better.

Overall, "From Crazy to Calm" is intended to be a helpful and encouraging book that can show you how to take small steps towards feeling better for yourself, and those you love, and help you realize that you can improve your mental health in natural and sustainable ways.

Disclaimer: We're not medical doctors - nor do we claim to be. We don't diagnose or prescribe. We recommend based on our education and knowledge. Each chapter stands alone as the personal experiences and expert opinion of the author. Each author takes responsibility and accountability for their own business. No claims are made on specific outcomes. Our goal is to open your eyes to alternatives that may be worth learning more about. Always talk to your doctor, especially if you have a diagnosis. Let's all be partners on your journey to finally feeling good NOW.

A BRIDGE TO HEALTH

Alternative health modalities serve as bridges, connecting the timeless wisdom of traditional health practices with the advancements and possibilities of whole health care.

In their harmonious embrace, these different modalities weave together the wisdom of ancient healing practices, passed down through generations, with the boundless potential offered by scientific advancements and technological innovations.

Together they form an intricate tapestry, where the threads of traditional knowledge and contemporary research intermingle, creating a holistic approach that honors the foundations of the past while embracing the possibilities of the future.

This bridge creates a holistic approach that embraces the best of both worlds, fostering a profound connection between mind, body, and spirit."

INTRODUCTION

"You're going to read or control my mind." Those words seemed comical to me as my hypnotherapy instructor told us we might come across people who actually think that's what a hypnotherapist does.

My hypnotherapy instructor said that there were many myths about what hypnosis was, and the stigma had been around for years. It didn't make sense to me. During the class, I witnessed so many amazing breakthroughs from those who had issues, false beliefs, and negative thoughts they had been trying to release for years. They hadn't been able to get to the root of these issues. It took hypnosis to open the subconscious to the conscious to release them, to guide them in their own healing from them and change their beliefs.

It was powerful to watch this transformation. I learned the science behind hypnosis. I became excited to share this with those I love and those whom I came in contact with.

When he warned us about what we might encounter, I chuckled, "Really? Control a mind? Read a mind? People actually thought this was true?"

"Hmm", could the words my instructor said to us actually be true? Was there actually so much stigma and myths around hypnosis?

As I headed out on my journey as a newly certified hypnotherapist, some were receptive; others looked at me with that deer-in-the-headlight stare, obviously feeling uncomfortable with the subject.

I attended my first Energy Healing Conference. I walked in, and I felt like I was home. I thought, "These are my people." It was so exciting and had so much great energy. Everything was new to me. I felt like a kid in a candy store. I wanted to learn all I could about this new world I had just stepped into.

With enthusiasm, I walked up to each practitioner and told them how excited I was to be there, that I had never been to something like this before, and I just wanted to know what they were doing. Their first question to me was, "Are you a practitioner?" I blurted out, "Yes, I'm a Certified Hypnotherapist."

Their reactions weren't what I had anticipated. They looked at me like I was "the devil." The words my instructor forewarned us, "You're going to read my mind or control my mind," were very apparent on their faces as they quickly changed the subject. Although they were kind, I could tell they were uncomfortable and wanted me nowhere near their booths.

After several of these same reactions, I stopped for a moment, and it caused me to chuckle. Here I was surrounded by practitioners who thought I was "woo, woo, and weird", yet they used crystals, stones, essential oils, and modalities like "Reiki," "Energy Code," "Intuitive Healing," "Healing Lights," "Muscle Testing," "Chakras." And, yet they thought I was the weird one?

I thought, "If I could have controlled anyone's mind, I would have wanted to control my daughters when they were teenagers." "If I could read anyone's mind, I would want to read my husband's.... I think."

As I walked through the event that day, I saw no hypnotherapists. I attended several classes. One, in particular, was taught by the event organizer. She was kind, outgoing, and fun. It was fabulous. She talked about energy in a way I had never heard of before. It opened my mind to the concept that "everything is energy." When she introduced her program, I was one of the first ones to sign up. I wanted to learn everything I could about energy. I also left the conference with a new goal. I would be one of the Energy Healing Conference's main speakers. Little did I know the obstacle that lay ahead of that goal.

I started taking her class. All this energy stuff started making sense to me. She is a natural promoter and cheerleader. She loves to connect people to each other. If she feels they can benefit from what you can teach them, she eagerly sends them to you. During class, she would say, "Are you a practitioner? If so, let me know, and I'll promote you on my website and events." I would eagerly say, "I'm a Certified Hypnotherapist." Silence. No acknowledgement, crickets. Nothing. I said this to her a couple of times with the same reaction. I realized that the owner of the largest Energy Healing Conference had the same false perspective of what hypnosis was. That is why there were no hypnotherapists at her event.

With this understanding, I realized it would take a lot more manifesting for my goal to become one of her main speakers to come true.

I realized at that moment there was a distinct line between hypnotherapists and energy healing practitioners. They wanted nothing to do with me.

Although hypnosis has been scientifically proven, there really was a stigma of myths surrounding hypnotherapy. I decided that it was ok. I would learn all I could about this other world called "energy healing" so I could increase the tools in my healing toolbox that I could use to help clients.

About a year and a half later, I learned about Amino Acid Therapy. I was so excited to share with anyone who would listen about what happens when the neurotransmitters in the brain (that produce your happy, calm, positive, feel-good chemicals) become depleted causing mental, emotional, and physical symptoms; and creating insatiable cravings, addictions, undesirable habits, and weight gain.

I wanted to share the knowledge that by feeding the brain - it's best food, a.k.a.- specific amino acids, I could help someone balance the brain; and reduce negative symptoms, cravings, addictions, and weight gain.

I ran into the event organizer, my now new friend, at a Christmas concert. She was eating a double scoop of ice cream. She asked what I was doing now. I excitedly told her I had learned about the brain, how to feed it, and how to reduce cravings such as sugar. She sheepishly continued to lick her double scoop ice cone when she told me she wanted to have a session with me.

It was after that meeting that she asked me if I'd ever thought of speaking. She asked me to be one of her speakers. So crazy! So excited! Of course, I said emphatically, "YES."

I later told her of my experience attending my first Energy Healing Conference, how I had written down that I wanted to become one of her speakers, and how I felt that she was against hypnosis. She chuckled when she told me I was right. Due to personal experiences in her past, she was afraid of hypnosis. She saw it as evil.

Luckily for me, during that year and a half, one of my hypnotherapy friends had also wanted to be one of her speakers. She refused until he offered her a free session, and she realized the power of hypnosis. He became one of her speakers several miles away from me. This opened the door for her to feel comfortable with hypnosis and allowed me to become one of her speakers. Thus, opening the door of energy healing meets hypnosis.

Oh, and those crazy energy healers I met at the first conference who thought I was woo woo, and I thought they were? I've worked with them, and they've worked with me. I've learned so many different modalities, which has made me a much better hypnotherapist. They've used my supplements, and many of them have added them to their own practice. I feel blessed to call them my dear friends.

Why this book? I know I am not the only one who has no clue about the power of energy healing, just like so many of you who may also have no knowledge of the power of alternative health options through energy healing, hypnotherapy, amino acids, etc.

This book is a simple read. I've brought together several of my favorite leading experts to help you see that there is a world of alternative health available to you. This doesn't mean you must throw everything you already know and feel about your health out the window. It's opening your eyes to energy healing and hypnotherapy.

This information may give you answers you've been looking for and haven't found in traditional health care. It's not one against the other. It's just options and looking at life a little differently.

Why? Life Matters.... YOU Matter.

"Gratitude:

A magnet for miracles."

Chapter 1:

Gratitude, Laughter, and Joy, Oh My!

By Carrie Verrocchio, MBA
CarrieVee

How do we reduce stress, increase productivity, and live with greater purpose and passion? The answer lies in gratitude, laughter, and joy. George Bernard Shaw has stated, "We don't stop playing because we grow old. We grow old because we stop playing." More play and more gratitude equal less chaos and more calm. So, are you ready to find more joy and peace in your life? If so, read on!

How tapped into your emotions are you? Do you allow yourself to laugh AND cry? Feel joy AND sadness? Are you able to ask why and know you will be okay - even while it seems like your life is falling apart?

1

Is it possible to feel sadness and laugh at the same time? Is it possible to feel gratitude while stress threatens to overwhelm you? Is it possible to laugh and cry at the same time? How important are laughter, joy, and gratitude?

Are you feeling off as you are reading this chapter? Maybe there is sadness in your life. Maybe a bit of trepidation. Is something in your life not turning out the way you thought it would? Perhaps you are feeling stressed over a situation you have no control over. Maybe you're already thinking about skipping this chapter because the thought of gratitude, laughter, and joy is so foreign in your life that it is almost insulting that I would even be writing about it.

After all, how is this crazy woman named CarrieVee going to convince you that gratitude can bring your life into focus for more laughter and more joy? And then she thinks she is going to convince you that all the laughter and joy will reduce stress, balance your hormones, make you smarter, increase your productivity, and bring success, too. CarrieVee has gone crazy.

Or has she?

How long do you think it takes to shift emotions and attitudes? It doesn't take long at all. **Emotions are affected by thoughts, feelings, and responses. Attitude is a choice. Happiness and Gratitude are decisions, and decisions require ACTION. Actions determine who you will BECOME. This chapter will focus on the actions of Gratitude, Laughter, and Joy.**

2

Gratitude

Let's begin with Gratitude, which is, our strongest foundation for more Laughter and Joy in our lives- and, therefore, more success and productivity. **In order to be truly successful, gratitude MUST be a part of your life.** It has been said that gratitude turns what we have into enough. When you complain about how things are, you invite more complaints into your life. When you practice gratitude, you invite more gratitude into your life. And when we **JOURNAL** our gratitude, we take it to an even higher level.

There are five reasons we want to journal our gratitude - ready?

1. It increases your PRODUCTIVITY. That may be reason enough for you to want to grab your journal and start jotting down the things you're grateful for. Here's what happens: Jot down some things you are grateful for, and BOOM, you automatically become more optimistic and start focusing on the positive rather than the negative. Then BOOM again - the optimism raises your energy, and - yep- BOOM again, and your productivity has skyrocketed. It's true. Next time you're feeling defeated, start journaling things that you are grateful for, then go back to the task at hand - I bet you may complete it in record time - simply by changing your focus from the negative to the positive.

2. It improves your SELF-ESTEEM. By expressing your gratitude, you are less likely to be resentful toward others. In other words, we stop comparing ourselves to everyone else around us. Studies show gratitude increases athletic performance, trust, and belief in yourself and your unique abilities, strengths, and gifts.

3. Gratitude also invites BETTER SLEEP. How? Spending a few minutes at night journaling a few things you are grateful for puts your mind on the positive as you fall asleep. Instead of falling asleep worrying or focusing on negativity, you fall asleep focused on gratitude. You are literally clearing your mind for a good night's sleep. I dare you to try this tonight.

4. It invites HAPPINESS into your life. Research shows us that individuals who journal their gratitude are more optimistic and feel better about their lives in general. They feel more positive emotions, appreciate their lives, are fully present in their lives, and build stronger relationships. This all translates into a much happier life!

5. It REDUCES STRESS. When you are grateful, you tend to take better care of yourself. In the long run, that means a healthier life. And that healthier life translates into the ability to better handle stress. In addition, science has shown that focusing on feelings of gratitude is a natural antidote to dealing with stress. It leaves you feeling more focused, grounded, and present - and more able to deal with what life throws at you.

When we put all that together: Gratitude makes you a happier you, a fitter you, and a better you.

So how do we go about beginning to journal our gratitude? Three Suggestions that we can do this right now: Get that paper and a pen. Time to write!

1. Be thankful for your life. Yes, with all of its craziness and hurt, be thankful for your life. In the unbearable pain and questions, be thankful for your life. **Take a moment to jot down a few ways to create a refreshing break for yourself.** A short walk, a dance in your kitchen, a cup of tea? **How can you create a 5-minute break just for you?** Take some time to breathe - deeply. Jot down some things you can be grateful for (food, a bed, children, a significant other, friends, a washer and dryer, your dog or cat?)

2. TELL SOMEONE YOU APPRECIATE THEM. Before this week is over, make a list of 30 people you are thankful for. Then once a day over the next 30 days, write a note to these people - and MAIL them. The point is actually to tell someone every single day that you appreciate them. **Your awareness that good DOES exist will increase your gratitude AND your appreciation for your life. It will help you see that despite the things that are going on in your life, you can be grateful.**

BONUS: Have some small cards made that simply say, "Thank you." Carry them with you when you want to show gratitude to someone who shows you kindness in a store, airport, restaurant, etc. Keep that gratitude at the forefront of your mind and life.

3. Begin a Gratitude Journal. Remember - What you focus on, you create MORE of. Focus on your problems, and you will create more problems. Focus on gratitude, and you create more gratitude. Get yourself a journal and begin each day with this prompt: "Today I am thankful for___" Then fill in the blank with **three** simple things you are grateful for. It can be as simple as toothpaste, toothbrush, or soap. Repeat this just before you go to bed. Keeping this gratitude journal will have a profound effect on your attitude and your life.

Try it right now. Take note of how the gratitude felt as you journaled things you are grateful for. Remember, gratitude is your foundation for more happiness and joy in your life. And that happiness and joy help you to reduce your stress - and deal with your stress. That happiness and joy, just like gratitude, helps to balance your hormones (which makes us more focused!). And it makes you smarter - simply by clearing your mind of negativity and giving you space to focus and learn.

In essence, choosing happiness (by choosing gratitude!) equals choosing success. Laughter and joy come before the success and not the other way around. When you start to laugh, that positive energy builds, and when that positive energy builds, you get greater ideas and more energy, and that equals more success. And the truth is this - you deserve success. It is out there for you. But you must first **choose** more happiness. More laughter. More joy. Success will follow.

But wait. Since when did happiness and laughter become a **choice**? Don't wait for a situation to be happy in order to laugh? Isn't that what you have always been taught? What if, despite any trial you go through, you choose to reframe the situation? Because the fact is, many times, if you are going to be happy and joyful, it's because you will have to make a considerable effort to do so.

Plain and simple, life isn't always going to go your way. And that is no excuse for being miserable. When you are choosing to be miserable, you are basically saying, "I give up my success, and I choose not to move forward." **You can choose to be positive, or you can choose to be negative, and both take energy. Choose wisely.**

What if you simply decided to create more laughter and joy in our lives despite your circumstances? What if you decided to build positive energy in your life? All that positive energy gives you access to greater ideas, more energy - and more success. You are not moving forward if you are stuck in a pit. And you can stay in the pit, or you can crawl out. It's your choice. Choose Wisely.

Abraham Lincoln has been credited with saying, "People are just about as happy as they make up their minds to be." We all have our trials and our scars. So why do some people remain in a pit of despair while others rise? The answer is simple (but not easy!). Those who rise to CHOOSE to do so by choosing gratitude, happiness, laughter, and joy - despite the heartache they are experiencing.

But CarrieVee - who has time for fun and happiness? We are BUSY people. Playtime, fun, and joy are a privilege afforded to those who are already successful. Right?

I used to think that way. Once the work is done and you have claimed success, THEN you have earned the right to take time for fun. You may think that having fun is something to feel guilty about. In the hustle of life, the things that make you happy are drowned out by all the noise, clutter, and daily demands and drama that close in on you.

Playtime, fun, happiness, joy, and laughter are what make us successful. Yet we often try to put them off until we ARE successful.

The problem is - it doesn't work that way.

The Science of choosing more fun, laughter, and joy are:

1. **Improved Relationships** - at work and in your personal life. Having fun with others helps build trust and develops communication. You connect more deeply when you incorporate more fun, laughter, and joy into your interactions with others. When companies incorporate time JUST to HAVE FUN, productivity skyrockets, and job satisfaction increases. Customers are happy. Retention rates are higher.

2. **Greater Profits** Having more fun (happiness and joy!) makes you smarter and more profitable. It improves your memory and concentration. **Happy, joyful, and fun activities introduce us to new ideas and concepts that lead to better self-directed learning, which leads to greater success - just for having more laughter and more fun.**

3. **Stress Reduction** - And reduced stress equals greater productivity and greater success.

4. **Balanced Hormones**. High-stress levels negatively affect our hormones -think cortisol. Stress also

negatively affects our endocrine systems, metabolic systems, and immune functions. And guess what happens when you're sick? You are not building your success. By consistently choosing happiness and joy and FUN - you can help balance out your hormone levels and strengthen our immune system - less time being sick and more time building success.

5. **Increased Energy**. More fun (happiness and joy!) makes you more youthful and increases your energy. Think about it, stress sucks the life out of us and makes us cranky and tired. Increased energy equals increased productivity and increased success.

So, get out there and have some FUN. Laugh! I dare you!

Still, got your pen and a journal? Good! Begin a list of ways YOU love incorporating laughter and joy into your life, and then CHOOSE to make time every day to laugh. Maybe it's dancing, playing a game, or walking the dog. Maybe it's painting or making candles. Maybe it's a funny movie. There are no rules here - just you choosing to have more fun in your life.

You choose not to be successful when you choose not to have fun.

Choose Gratitude. Choose Happiness. Choose Success.

Life is Short, my friends. Choose Wisely.

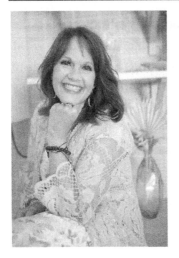

About the Author:
CarrieVee (Verrocchio) MBA

CarrieVee (Verrocchio) MBA, International Speaker and Author, Podcast Host, and Certified Transformation, Forgiveness, and Grief Coach, helps those who have forgotten how to dream, how to overcome their excuses and live the lives they were created to live.

She is the founder of the Radical Empowerment Method - a program designed to walk people through the exact method she used to move from a life of feeling invisible to a life of empowered success and action.

She is a Toastmasters Semi-Finalist in the 2020 World Championship of Speaking, as well as a keynote speaker for Toastmasters. She has been featured in multiple media outlets and has spoken on stage to thousands of men and women.

With Gratitude, Laughter, and Joy!

CarrieVee (Verrocchio)

International Speaker and Trainer, Podcast Host, Best Selling Author, Certified Transformation, Forgiveness, and REBT Coach, Bella Vita, LLC

607-760-8401 www.coachcarriev.com
carriev@coachcarriev.com

Life is Short - Choose Wisely®

SCAN QR CODE: Step into your big life freebie.

"Muscle testing:

The body's whisper of wisdom."

Chapter 2:

What is Muscle Testing and How to Use It

By Pamela Tolman

hat is muscle testing? Muscle testing is a technique that uses the meridians with some of the major organs and the muscles in the body to receive answers about the body, mind, and spirit. It can be used to determine how one is performing emotionally, mentally, and physically. It is a means to uncover the unconscious beliefs that one holds deep within the mind and the body.

We have the belief systems that were given to us, some that we took on ourselves, and some that were passed down to us through the generations. When we have gone through traumas or other issues, and we come to the conclusion that we have dealt with them and they no longer affect us, it may amaze you how many times, I have proven that thought wrong through the use of muscle testing.

Muscle testing is a form of biofeedback. It takes place when a particular muscle is in a contracted state. While the muscle is in this stiffened state, slight pressure is applied. If the muscle remains locked, it is considered to give positive feedback. However, if the muscle weakens, it is then considered to be expressing negative feedback.

Here is an example. If I were working with a client, I would ask them to hold their arm out straight and make it stiff like a board. Then I would show them what it would feel like as I applied about two pounds of pressure to their arm. The next step would be to have the client state his or her name, "my name is____" after their name is stated, pressure would be applied to the hand or wrist area. The arm should remain in the locked position or, in other words, straight and strong.

Next, the client would state a false statement, after which slight pressure to the hand or wrist would be applied. With the false statement, there should be a weakness in the arm that allows it to be pushed down. Remember it is important to use the same amount of pressure both times. It is not a challenge to see who is stronger; instead, it is to apply just enough pressure that there is a weakness in the arm. The body will always know what is true and what is false. Too many times, you tell yourself that you are okay when it really isn't true. That falsehood can cause major disruption in your life.

When your body is in harmony and balance, the muscles are strong and in sync. However, when there is a feeling of fear, pain, self-doubt, and being in a poor mental state, there is disharmony in the body, and it reacts with weakness. When you believe and agree to something subconsciously, your muscles will perform with strength, whereas if your subconscious mind disagrees and is negative, then the muscles will become weak. Muscle testing can be used as a bridge between the conscious and the subconscious mind. Just because you consciously believe something to be correct or good for you doesn't mean that the subconscious mind agrees with it.

The subconscious mind is what runs us, not the conscious mind; the conscious mind can and will trick us into believing, whereas the subconscious mind will never lie to us. If you want the deep truth, go to the subconscious for the answers.

Muscle testing can be used to increase your own self-awareness. Would you like to know how certain foods, supplements, or even your environment influence you? How about identifying your limiting beliefs and the emotions that restrict you from making positive changes in your personal life?

One of the benefits of using muscle testing is that you have all the equipment you need with you at all times in your body. Also, you can use it anywhere and at any time.

There are several ways to muscle test. Here are a few of my favorite ways.

15

1. Sway- the easiest for my clients to learn. When you first begin, stand with your feet together, eyes closed. Having your eyes closed takes out any distractions that might be in front of you. If you begin with your feet close together, then you will be able to feel even the slightest movement. Later as you practice more and become more accustomed to the feel, you can stand with your feet shoulder-width apart.

With eyes closed and feet together, ask your body to show you a "yes" answer; at this point, you should begin to feel a slight pull forward. Then you can ask the body to show you a "no" answer; here, you should feel a slight pull back. The forward motion is one of being positive or truthful, whereas a backward motion represents a negative or false answer. After you have established the yes and no motion, it is time to start asking the body questions.

Start with something simple like "My name is____" stating your name. Now if you state your name and you receive a "no" answer, it could be because you are using a nickname and not your given name, so try again using your given name. Once you have received a positive answer, it is time to test a false statement. So again, you could say, "My name is ____," only this time use a fake name. To this, the body should move in a backward motion showing you that the statement is untrue.

Now you can start asking the more important questions that are on your mind. You might ask if a certain food or supplement is right for you. You may want to know what is holding you back from moving forward in life or letting go of something in the past.

The more intense the question, the deeper you must go. It is best to have help at this time from someone that is trained in asking the proper questions in the right way in order to receive the answers that are waiting for you.

If you are having trouble establishing true and false answers, there are a few things to consider. Are you standing in your own way? Have a little faith in yourself, get out of your own way, and believe you will receive the correct answers.

Interference? Things you might check; Jewelry worn by you or your muscle tester - Eyeglasses -Perfume -Cologne. To overcome those interferences, just remove glasses or jewelry, or wash off cologne or perfume and try again. Practice is important, don't give up; you will get it. Just keep going and believe in yourself.

2. Intertwined fingers method. With this, you will touch the thumb and middle finger of one hand together, so it looks like an 'O' with the rest of your fingers facing upward. Then place the middle finger of the opposite hand through the ring and touch the thumb. This forms a link, as you would see on a chain. Then decide which hand will be used as the strength and which one will be used as the release.

To make sure you're in tune with your body, even when you've had many years of experience, ask your body this simple question to begin, 'show me a YES answer' and if the fingers hold strong, that's your YES answer. Then ask, 'show me a NO answer' and if one set of fingers goes weak to release the link, that's how you know your NO answer. Practice until you feel confident that you are receiving the correct answers.

It is important to understand that you are working with the body's energy system. Therefore, you need to recognize when you are in the way. Are you always getting a yes answer to a question that you want the answer to be yes to?

Let me explain I once worked with a young lady that had found out she was going to have a baby; she was so excited and wanted to know if she would be having a girl or a boy. First, I told her she would have to wait for a few months before she could take the test. There are several reasons for this, which are too extensive for this chapter, so be sure to check out my book.

She returned at a later date, so excited to tell me she had tested, and she was going to have the baby girl she had hoped for. It is not for me to tell a person that they are wrong. However, I did ask her certain questions about her testing. One question I asked was, "Were you hoping or thinking that the test would be a yes for a girl?" When she told me that she was really hoping for a girl, I explained how the force of energy works.

In her case, she really wanted a baby girl; she had been hoping for a girl from the time she found out she was pregnant, so even though she was trying not to think about it during the muscle testing, that is exactly what she was thinking about. Therefore, she was influencing the energy to give her the answer she was looking for. In order to receive a truthful answer, you must remove yourself completely from the force field of energy. You must trust yourself enough to move over and get out of the way so that the life force energy can perform in the way that you are asking it to. If you are not able to get out of the way and become unattached to the answers you receive, you may not receive the correct answers.

- When asking, make an affirmative statement that will allow for a clear and more precise answer. For example: Using the statement "Should I make this change in my life?" You may believe that you are ready to make the changes in your life; however, by using the word "should," you may be led to internal conflicts with what you desire and what your true readiness is in moving forward. You may want to change the statement to one such as "I am ready to make this change in my life!"

Now is the time to jump in, trust yourself, get out of your way, and start using muscle testing to improve your life. I believe in YOU!

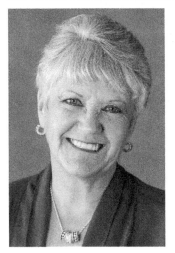

About the Author
Pamela Tolman,

Pam Tolman is a Master Certified Clinical Hypnotherapist. She began almost 30 years ago after a diagnosis of multiple sclerosis.

After this life-changing diagnosis, she focused on using hypnotherapy, meditation, and other techniques, to help her control her condition.

This change ignited a desire in her to share what she had learned to help others. Pam has spent thousands of hours educating herself, teaching others, and speaking to groups at colleges and conferences in NV, UT, WY, ID, and MT.

She owns a hypnotherapy practice and school. She is a published author of the book Hypnosis for Faster Pain Relief. Pam is an international speaker.

She considers it her personal mission to help others to release the bonds of addiction, excess weight, chronic pain, grief, anxiety, and day-to-day stress. She helps with feelings of temporomandibular joints (TMJ), PTSD, sleep disorders, and sports.

On a couple of special occasions, Pam has helped friends with hypnobirthing. On the other side of that, she has had the opportunity to be with a family taking them through the transition as their loved one left this life for a new journey.

In her work as a clinical hypnotherapist. Pam is passionate about strengthening individuals and families by tailoring the different techniques to their needs. Thus, ensuring that each and every day is truly seen as the gift it is meant to be. Pam does more than survive; She "THRIVES," and so can you!

 **SCAN QR CODE to**
pamshealthandhealing.com
hypnotekniq@yahoo.com
pam@pamshealthandhealing.com
Facebook – Pam's Health and Healing

Phone: 307-887-0138

"Nourish your brain,

unleash your potential."

Chapter 3:

Amino Acids Create Brain Health

By Shelly Jo Spinden Wahlstrom

*S*ix words, six simple words changed my life. How could six words change my life? My fifteen-year-old daughter came to me in tears and cried, "Mom, I'm tired of being a doctor's science project!" Here are those six words "I JUST WANT TO FEEL NORMAL!" My heart sank.

Have you ever felt helpless and hopeless? This is how I felt at that moment. I had failed my daughter, yet we had done everything we thought was right for her.

At age six, my daughter was diagnosed with anxiety. "It's just a chemical in the brain," said the school counselor. "All you have to do is get her on an inexpensive medication and she'll be fine." We did that. We did what all parents did, at the time. We got her on meds and into counseling and assumed she would be just fine.

When she made that statement, the realization that she wasn't fine hurt my heart. Unfortunately, she turned to drugs and alcohol "just to feel normal." This put us on a scary journey. Addiction didn't make any sense to me. I thought I could ground her or love her enough. Obviously, I'm sure you can figure out how these approaches didn't work.

When "we" graduated from high school. Notice the "we." It took a lot to get her to graduate. If you've ever had a child who struggles, you understand the "we." We put her in a rehab program. We paid thousands of dollars to help her get clear. Thirty days later, she did come out clean from marijuana and alcohol. However, she came out addicted to sugar, caffeine, and tobacco.

I thought we had won the fight over addiction. Little did I know that it was only the beginning. Thirty days later, she was introduced to meth. She became instantly addicted. Meth is the drug of the devil. It changes every part of you. I was instantly thrown into excessive fear and felt powerless.

Each day I lived in fear that she would hurt me, kill someone, kill herself or end up in jail. The first time she ended up in jail, I was actually relieved. I could breathe and sleep knowing where she was and that she was safe. In my naivety, I thought this was the turning point. She had the desire to change her life. I thought she would. I watched her stay clean for about six months, relapse, and end up in jail. It didn't make any sense to me.

"I DON'T WANT TO LOSE MY DAUGHTER!" were the words I yelled when the only thing I could think of was to pray. God, please help my daughter. Please help me find answers.

This put me on a journey to find out what I didn't understand about the brain and addiction. Now at this point, you may be thinking, "Wait, I'm not a hardcore addict. What does this have to do with me?"

Do you, your child, teen, or other loved ones, struggle with one or many feelings or frustrations above or experiences below?

- Anxiety, depression, OCD, perfection, ruminating negative thoughts, low self-esteem, anger.
- Lack of energy, focus, motivation, or sleep.
- STRESS, overwhelmed, uptight.
- Grief, sensitive to emotional or physical pain, self-harm (cutting, nail-biting, hair pulling, etc.)

When feeling this way, do you or your loved one turn to something listed below to feel better?

- Sugar, Starches, Caffeine, Aspartame, Chocolate
- Drugs - legal or illegal
- Alcohol
- Behaviors: too much gaming, social media, shopping, gambling, pornography, work.

If you answer yes to any of these questions, then I'm talking to you. At first, when I learned about these tools, I became angry. "Why hadn't I heard about these options when my daughter was six? At six, she wasn't an addict. Had I known this information when she was six, she may not have turned to drugs and alcohol at age fifteen?" I decided then that this information needs to get out so that I can help that mother who has a child struggling, the teenager struggling with life attached to their phone; or the adult "just white-knuckling it".

What does this look like? **FEED YOUR BRAIN - CHANGE YOUR LIFE, Take Control of Your Brain, Body, and Emotions.** This is also the title of my bestselling book sold on Amazon.

- **Feed Your Brain** - Brain Food.
- **Feed Your Body Nutrition.** There's a connection between the brain and body when it comes to mental health. What you eat matters.
- **Feed and change your thoughts through Hypnotherapy/Hypnosis.** You can read more about this in **Chapter 13 of this book.**

WHAT ARE NEUROTRANSMITTERS

In the brain, you have Neurotransmitters. These are your "Happy, Calm, Positive, Feel Good" chemicals. When they are firing, they are wonderful. When they are not, then they're not. They can cause all the feelings listed above and more. Our brains like to live in homeostasis (balance). When we feel these feelings, our brain wants something to feel better and turns to something that can give it the easiest and fastest feelings. It's looking for sugar, starches, drugs, alcohol, or behaviors.

HOW DO NEUROTRANSMITTERS BECOME DEPLETED

- A child born with less of them.
- Stress
- Lifestyle
- Diet
- Toxins
- The body doesn't produce enough specific amino acids to feed Neurotransmitters.
- Sixty Percent of people over the age of 40
- Living in a perfectly imperfect body with a perfectly imperfect brain in other words, there's no real way to say why they've become depleted.

NEUROTRANSMITTERS AND HOW THEY MAKE YOU FEEL

Feeding the brain-specific brain food can help raise and balance the neurotransmitters, which will then help to reduce feelings. That, in turn, helps reduce cravings, addictions, and behaviors.

What are Neurotransmitters, and how do they make you feel when they are firing correctly?

- **SEROTONIN: Positive mind, confidence, flexibility, humor**
- **DOPAMINE: Energy, focus, drive, concentration**
- **GABA: Physically able to relax.**
- **ENDORPHINS: Happy**

27

HOW TO BOOST NEUROTRANSMITTERS

1. Exercise
2. Spend Time in Nature
3. Nutrition - Protein, Omega 3
4. Meditation
5. Gratitude
6. Essential Oils - Bergamot, Lavender, Lemon
7. Goal Achievement
8. Happy Memories
9. Novelty
10. Therapy

(https://www.goodtherapy.org/blog/10-ways-to-boost-dopamine-and-serotonin-naturally-1212177)

What's the difference between boosting and balancing? Boosting is to temporarily boost the neurotransmitter to help you feel better for a small amount of time. Balancing and raising is by feeding the neurotransmitters what they already use, which is either created in the body or by a supplement to get them from a depleted state to firing with the idea that eventually, once they are no longer depleted, they may be able to fire without taking a supplement for the rest of your life. This time period is different for everyone. It may be a month to a year or more, depending on how long they've been depleted.

HOW TO FEED, BALANCE, AND RAISE NEUROTRANSMITTERS NATURALLY

- **SEROTONIN - 5-HTP POSITIVE MIND®, L-TRYPTOPHAN POSITIVE SLEEP®**

- **DOPAMINE - L-TYROSINE ENERGY BOOSTER®**
- **GABA - GABA CHILL®**
- **ENDORPHINS - DLPA HAPPY®**

You may be able to figure out which of your neurotransmitters may be depleted and which amino acid may be your answers by going to hypnoaminos.com and taking the quiz "Could Amino Acids Be YOUR Missing Link?" (See the link in my bio following this chapter).

One other thing to think about when it comes to mental health is the role blood sugar plays.

In the brain, you have what's called the "Prefrontal Cortex." It's the brain's cognitive thought process. It's your reasoning, judgment, and willpower. When it's functioning properly, it also is a tool to help someone struggling with cravings and addiction stay clean. It helps you think through your choices and consequences. "If I make this choice, this will be the outcome or consequence, good or bad."

When we're eating too much sugar, starches; drinking too much alcohol; fasting, starving, or skipping meals; it shuts off the Prefrontal Cortex and puts us into a hypoglycemic state where we become irritable and irrational. Irritable is that "hangry" feeling where suddenly your brain becomes foggy, your brain takes you hostage and tells you "GIVE ME WHAT I WANT NOW!!!" That may be sugar. This causes us to want to find anything that will feed it.

Instantly by feeding sugar, it spikes the blood sugar; which then the body increases insulin; which causes blood sugar to drop; which causes the body to increase adrenaline which causes sugar craving; And, then puts you on a roller coaster of blood sugar raising and dropping.

Alcohol drunk on an empty stomach may cause blood sugar to drop dramatically too low, which also puts you on this roller coaster.

One last thing about blood sugar. Did you know that using brain energy for work, school, studying, and exercise reduces glutamine and glucose in your body, which can also put you on this roller coaster?

HOW TO KEEP BLOOD SUGAR BALANCED

1. Eat 20-30 grams of protein 3-4 times a day.

2. **L-GLUTAMINE CRAVING BE GONE®** - L-Glutamine feeds every cell in your body. It also may help heal the mucus membrane of your stomach.

You can read more about each of the Neurotransmitters, amino acids, and nutrition in my book **FEED YOUR BRAIN CHANGE YOUR LIFE. Take Control of Your Brain, Body, and Emotions** Sold on Amazon. https://amzn.to/3ovJZTd

I've seen miracles with people when they start taking amino acid supplements. However, they're not magic. If you purchase them and don't take them, they're just pretty supplements sitting on your shelf. That, my friend, seems like a waste of money to me.

It warms my heart when I hear things like this from those whom this information has changed their lives:

"Shelly Jo really knows her products and has such passion for helping others. Her products have changed mine and my children's life forever! Love all the products and her book.

Thanks, Shelly Jo, for doing the thing you were uniquely created to do! You ROCK!" - Amy

"I am new to learning about amino acids and ordered them to get my 15-year-old some benefits she desperately needs. Already I see a calmer energy and within the first week she was sleeping better and telling me without me asking her." - Cathy

Take a moment to take care of yourself or those you love. These may be answers you've never heard of before. As I said before, I wish I had known these answers when my daughter was six. **Now I want you to know about them so you can take control of your brain, body, and emotions and LIVE BOLDLY.**

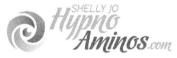

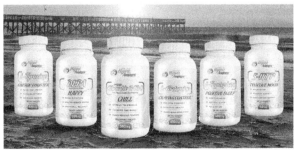

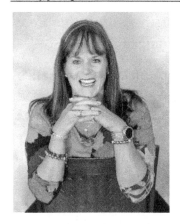

About the Author
Shelly Jo Spinden Wahlstrom, CHT, CRNC

Shelly Jo aka "The Amino Acid Lady and Hypnotherapist - is a Certified Hypnotherapist, Certified Addiction, Recovery, and Mental Health Nutrition Coach.

She is currently working on her Doctorate in Metaphysics from the University of Sedona in AZ.

Shelly Jo is the Owner of Shelly Jo Hypno Aminos Nutrition - a.k.a. brain food (voted - Top 25 Coolest Things Made in Utah - Best Natural Products - Standard Examiners - Best of Northern Utah - Best Hypnotherapy Service).

She is a Best-Selling Author - "Feed Your Brain, Change Your Life - Take Control of Your Brain, Body, and Emotions."

She is an International Speaker and Presenter. She teaches a Basic Amino Acid & Nutrition Course for practitioners interested in adding amino acids and nutrition to their practice.

Shelly Jo is the Chairperson of the Alliance for Addiction Solutions.

She lives in Utah with her husband, three amazing daughters and son-laws and favorite eleven grandchildren.

She is an avid skier, dancer, and player with grandchildren. Her favorite name is "Grama Shelly."

 SCAN QR CODE: Quiz, Website, to Connect:

Hypnoaminos.com

801-643-3211

shellyjo@hypnoaminos.com

linktr.ee/shellyjohypno

Could Amino Acids Be YOUR Missing Link

"Healing at Your Fingertips."

Chapter 4:

Zero-Point Meridian Technique
Shift Your Mood in Five Minutes or Less

By Cristine Price, Ph.D., CMHC

Have you regretted your actions after being emotionally triggered? Maybe, like many of us, you've resorted to overeating, oversleeping, or verbally attacking a stranger, or, even worse, a loved one. Reactions can happen even to those who've been in therapy for a while, even those who have a strong support system, and even those who are trusted in leadership roles. Negative emotions are the most common low-frequency challenges faced by the best of us.

After decades of providing professional therapy, Cristine Price, Ph.D., has developed an efficient and effective tool, shown to dramatically decrease emotionality in only five minutes. Most mental health therapists aren't even aware of the technique, but Cristine has been using it for over twenty years with success. Like any self-help tool, it isn't designed to replace professional or medical support. However, it can certainly aid you at the moment. As you follow the process, you are taking responsibility for your own mental and emotional well-being as well as those in your environment who your emotions can positively impact. Before we look at the technique, let's first assess emotional levels and patterns.

What is a SUD?

Subjective Units of Distress (or SUD) score is a rating of emotional distress on a 1-10 scale.

A SUD of 10 is the most intense, and a SUD of 1 is the opposite or the lowest level of distress. A SUD of 7 or higher would likely be considered anxiety. SUDs around 4-6 may be described as stress.

SUD scores are used in therapies for trauma or intense emotions, such as EMDR (Eye Movement Desensitization Reprocessing) and Brain spotting, (which is another neurological-emotional technique utilizing eye movement).

Rating emotional intensity is subjective. It is up to each person to determine what 10 feels like. For some, it is a full panic attack, and for others, it's intense discomfort. Rating the SUD level before using the technique allows for a baseline to be reassessed later. Mental health clients often report being between SUD=4 to SUD=8 most of the time. If you rate yourself at a SUD=9 or 10, please consider involving a professional or certified practitioner to support your process directly.

The long-term goal in using any technique for reducing stress would be to stop and interrupt the pattern before SUDs climb too high. Success requires self-awareness and self-discipline to interrupt the pattern. Your first goal may be to assess your SUDs frequently throughout the day and set an intention to stop and use the five-minute technique when your stress reaches a certain point, such as SUD=6.

Self-Awareness Assignments:

1. What is your current daily range of SUDs? How high does your stress or anxiety reach? How low does your score reach with relaxation or other stress-reduction techniques?
2. What percentage of the time are you over SUD=5? Gathering this baseline level can be very helpful as you continue.

What's Your Trigger?

Sometimes you run around with stress or anxiety and don't take the time to identify what sets you off. Noticing stressors allows for more proactive strategies. Which triggers are you affected by? Being specific is helpful in identifying and addressing stress levels.

- Running late
- Driving stress
- Time scarcity
- Financial scarcity

- Worrying about the health (or _____) of someone close
- Feeling powerless over a teenager's (or significant other's) behavior
- Getting in an argument with _____
- Pressures at work
- Not enough support

1. Now, pick one specific trigger that raises your stress. What stressor would you like to neutralize?
2. How high would you rate the Subjective Units of Distress with the specific stressor? SUD=_____

The Five-Minute Technique

This process is one part of the complete Zero-Point Meridian Technique. In this brief method, we will tap on one of nine total meridian points. These meridian points fit into an algorithm based on Traditional Chinese Medicine. In order to release emotions from both the mind and the vital body, we will use a combination of stimulating and calming the meridian point.

The full method explains the quantum nature of the Zero-point field as a way to reset the meridians.

For the brief method, we will keep it simple and just use an affirmation to support alignment or

"reset" the meridian.

The Meridian Point:

The point we will reset for the five-minute version is part of the small intestine meridian, located on the side of the palm. Simply tap the side of the dominant hand on the non-dominant palm or fingers as if "karate chopping."

The Zero-Point Meridian Technique has its roots in Emotional Freedom Technique (EFT). Cristine was fully trained in the original EFT in 2003 before spending a decade developing what her practitioners continue to affirm is a very different and unique method. One enhancement Cristine made was with Gary Craig's original Set-Up Statement. One of her first practitioners, Kolae Perkins, renamed it the "Alignment Statement" after discovering it aligned the energy body for the remaining process.

The Alignment Statement combined with the small intestine meridian makes up the Five-Minute Technique: Begin by acknowledging the problem and then align the meridian with a new, high-frequency intention. Choose from two optional endings:

A) "I love and accept myself completely, with Infinite Love and Gratitude, I release and forgive."

B) "I allow myself to be filled with infinite love and gratitude." Decide which feels best for you or applies to the situation.

C) **"Even though I _____ (have this problem), I love and accept myself completely, with Infinite Love and Gratitude I release and forgive." Or I allow myself to be filled with Infinite Love and Gratitude.**

39

1. Using the specific trigger above, fill in the blank of the Alignment Statement.
2. Tap on the small intestine meridian (karate chop point) while reading the statement aloud.
3. Hold the side of the palm while inhaling and exhaling completely.
4. Repeat the process two more times. You can keep the original statement or adjust it as needed.
5. Re-rate your SUD score.

Examples of Alignment Statements:

You may find it useful to use metaphors or adjectives that get to the root, for example, feeling trapped, blocked, or overwhelmed. Here are a few examples:

- Even though I have a chronic scarcity of money, I love and accept myself completely; with Infinite Love and Gratitude, I release and forgive.
- Even though I am paralyzed by low self-esteem, I allow myself to be filled with Infinite Love and Gratitude. Even though I am under pressure at work, I love and accept myself completely with Infinite Love and Gratitude; I release and forgive.
- Even though I am powerless over Joe's decisions, I love and accept myself completely; with Infinite Love and Gratitude, I release and forgive.
- Even though I am overwhelmed by anxiety, I allow myself to be filled with Infinite Love and Gratitude.

Your energy matters. It matters to your loved ones, your own well-being, your responsibilities, and even to random strangers. Your energy creates a ripple that can be positive or negative. Thank you for making it positive. To maximize the impact of this powerful technique, you'll want to use it daily if possible.

Daily Impact:

1) For at least a week, choose to use the Alignment Statement daily on a single situation or adapt the situation as needed. You may find that the problem you start with is resolved in a few days. Consider chronic patterns, images, and metaphors in your problem statement.

2) Rate your SUD range daily over the week. See if it adjusts from your baseline levels.

3) Also rate your SUD scores before and after using the Five-minute Technique that day.

	Day 1	Day 2	Day 3	Day 4	Day 5	Day 6	Day 7
SUD Range							
SUD before & after EFT							

Congratulations on learning and practicing this technique so you can show up in a more emotionally intelligent state for others. If you are looking for support with the process or the full technique, please

check our list of certified EFT practitioners. They can work with you using the full four-part Complete EFT Method. If you liked the five-minute process, you'd love the full experience that much more. Go to ConsciousCommUnity.college for information.

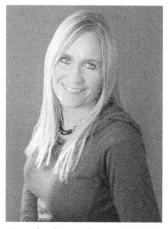

About the Author
Cristine Price, Ph.D., CMHC

Dr. Cristine Price began her career in the early 1990s as a Substance Abuse Counselor. Her own recovery in 1988 inspired her career path. She went on to get a Master's Degree in Psychology from Utah State University and a Doctorate in Natural Medicine from Quantum University.

She spent ten years in Davis School District as a School Psychologist, where she specialized in Emotional Disorders. Cristine discovered Emotional Freedom Technique in 2003 through Carol Tuttle, RET. She immediately completed basic and advanced training with Gary Craig. She discovered how quickly the technique worked with children, soothing their emotional reactions, getting them back to class, or allowing them to problem-solve and return to rational thinking. However, Cristine realized private practice was a more suitable setting for Energy Psychology.

Cristine began her career as an Integrative Mental Health Counselor in 2007, first working with an agency in Logan, Utah, and then establishing her own private practice. In 2015 she began her doctoral program in Natural Medicine, which validated what she'd already found, that the vital body is full of information necessary for comprehensive solutions. She has worked with the chakras and meridians for over two decades, along with the mind and emotions.

Since receiving her Ph.D. in 2020, Cristine has established herself as an Integrative Mental Health Consultant, bringing conscious solutions to practitioners, rehabs, and mental health providers. She has certified over thirty practitioners in Zero-Point Meridian Technique, formerly known as The Complete EFT Method. Her trainees' results consistently exceed those of mental health therapies such as EMDR for reducing stress and anxiety in sessions. In 2022, she married her soul mate and recovery partner, Todd E. Hull, inspiring the fictional series she'll soon release as Author Cristine Hull.

 **SCAN QR CODE Liberation Transformation Training**

More information about Cristine, along with the bookstore and the free ARISE Summit Series, can be found at: www.cristineprice.com or ConsciousCommUnity.college.

"Chakras:

Energy centers illuminating

the path within."

Chapter 5:

Calm Outweighs the Chaos
Through the Chakras

By Jerica Church

C*haos... Chaos happens when the body is out of alignment with itself spiritually, physically, and emotionally. What most people don't know is you have another system that can and will help you balance your chaos. I call it the electrical system. Your electric system is your chakras and meridians, and the purpose of these functions is to help your spiritual, physical, and emotional systems communicate.*

Think of this like a car; your spiritual part of yourself is the transmission, your physical part of yourself is the motor, and your emotional part of yourself is the radiator. Without the wires connection between all three functions, your car cannot properly run. A car depends on these main functions to move. Without proper communication, the car simply cannot move, or you could bust the motor, blow the radiator blow, or slip a gear. Your chakra system is the communication piece between our systems, and this work is what I am passionate about.

Hi! I'm Jerica Church, and I've been known as a guru in chakra work. I am passionate about teaching how chakras and holistic health modalities can truly make your life a little easier. The chaos never truly goes away; however, the calm will outweigh the chaos. In this chapter, I will go into each chakra and simply express what I have learned about each one. Now, keep in mind that there is so much that goes into each one I couldn't possibly share everything; however, I will do my best to give you a little taste.

Before we get into them, let me start by saying what chakras really are. They are energy. Everything is energy; we are taught that by Albert Einstein. It is science that we are literally energy, so with that being said, wouldn't it make sense to have balls of energy that help us in our everyday life? Chakras are balls, also known as disks of energy, that rotate in our bodies. There are over 230 chakras; however, we mostly talk about the main 7. Each of the main 7 has a function that helps us in our everyday lives.

The Root Chakra: Think of your root chakra as your basic needs are located at the base of your spine down to your feet. You must have shelter, food, and water to survive. The root chakra is all these things for your body. It's for safety and security. You will start thriving in your success when you begin to align with this chakra because

47

this is where manifestation in career and abundance in money shows up. Ground yourself daily and install the inspiration that you feel into your everyday day life by creating a plan and taking one step at a time.

The Sacral Chakra: Your sacral is your power! Located around your sacred parts (your creation space below the belt). In this space, you discover your passions and the importance of intimacy with yourself and your partner if/and when you enter into that phase. When you are able to balance creativity and intimacy, you begin to see a shift in your excitement in life.

The Solar Plexus Chakra: This chakra function is all about how we feel about ourselves. located from the navel to the breast. Did you know the majority of almost all people who struggle with self-esteem have tummy issues? There is a direct correlation, based on the intensity, between the stomach issues with how much you dislike yourself. We are taught that 90% of our physical pains are emotional. A great read is "Feelings Buried Alive Never Die." by Karol Kuhn Truman. This book talks about how that works. The truth is nobody can hate you with the intensity that you can hate yourself. Conversely, nobody can love you with the intensity that you can love yourself. That is why it is extremely important to release the thoughts society tells us we should be and learn to enjoy ourselves.

The Heart Chakra: It does just like it sounds. The heart is where our relationships with friends, family, and all loved ones are stored. Our heart is our leading chakra. This is where we love with our fullest potential, and our

48

humanity comes from. The majority of my clients have blocked energy from grief and sadness and stored them in their heart chakra. That can cause breakdowns, emotional distress, numbness, and more when we aren't able to process these emotions. Like all chakras, when we are able to process these emotions, we are able to feel calmer and less chaotic. I like to say this "A heart-balancing meditation a day keeps the doctor away."

The Throat Chakra: Located where your throat is! This chakra is all about speaking up for yourself. Of course, there is a high and low for each chakra. Some people might talk too much, and others might not talk enough. There is balance when you're living in your authentic self, and that looks different for everyone.

The 3rd Eye Chakra" a.k.a The Pineal Gland": Also known as your inner woo! This is located in the middle of your forehead between your eyes and the surrounding space. It has to do with our spiritual gifts and developing a deeper knowledge of the world around us. Your intuition and those little thoughts you have prompting you in different directions are coming from your 3rd eye.

The Crown Chakra: Located at the top of your head is where we connect with our spirituality. It doesn't matter what that is; what matters is that you believe in something. It can be God, the universe, Mother Nature, the highest self, the spirit, all of these, or maybe something else. It can literally be anything. What matters is you know you have a purpose and that you are here for a reason. When you are able to deepen that bond, you find your inspiration and flow of life becoming more in alignment.

Your healing journey is never truly over. Once you're dedicated to that path, you will always be looking to be one step better to become your highest self and become your highest potential. The chakras are a really great place to start if you are new to the energy world. It's also a great place to deepen when you are looking for that next level.

I began all of this work when I was at my deepest point during my first year of marriage. It was a whirlwind of pain, trauma, and loss that ended with a beautiful baby girl and postpartum depression. To this day, I believe our daughter saved our marriage, saved my husband's life, and she saved me. She gave me the desire to be better and want more in life.

I began looking for ways to help with my depression and ran into multiple modalities. I found the most healing for myself through the chakras, and to this day, as I learn more and grow, I will never regret the hard work and pain we went through to get to where we are today. And while we still have struggles and are still gifted with trials, I always return back to the chakras when I start feeling the chaos come back. I have been doing this for so long that I can truly say the chakras and chakra work have and still do help me in my everyday life. I never imagined myself buying crystals or even selling them, and now through this work, I have created a career and passion for myself and my family. I've gotten to the point where I love life, I love what I do, and I love sharing it all.

The last thing I will leave you with is you can change. Humans are designed to change and adapt. You can live a happier, healthy, and more fulfilled life.

So, if you feel you're not there yet now is your time to go find it. It is never too late, and it's never too early. You can do whatever it is that you set your mind to. All you need is a little love and a lot of passion.

Xoxo, Jerica Church.

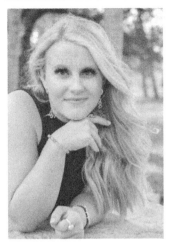

About the Author:
Jerica Church

Jerica and her husband currently own a holistic health shop and wellness center called All Things Holistic.

Jerica's main goal is to help educate about the woo world. Why is she passionate about chakras?

She is passionate about spreading the word on mental health and suicide awareness.

Her goal in life is to help people feel worthy of a life they can love.

She is known as the chakra guru. She speaks on many stages, teaches classes on crystals, chakras, and color therapy, and offers sound baths. She also offers cacao ceremonies and so many other healthy living modalities.

Her favorite thing is offering educational retreats. She hosts both domestic and international retreats in places such as Lake Tahoe, NV; Jackson Hole, WY; Huntsville, UT; Costa Rica; and Hawaii (just to name a few). Check out her website for future events.

Jerica is Certified in

- Certified in Chakra Basics 1 & 2
- Cacao Ceremonies
- Sound Baths
- Speaking on Self-Worth, Suicide & Depression Awareness.

Services include:

- Body Relaxation Sessions
- Certified Reiki & Reflexology
- Speaking on Chakras, crystals, and anything holistic
- Domestic and international retreats
- Online - 7-Week Chakra Class
- Shop in-person or online

Join the tribe:

- **by following her on Instagram: Jerica.Church**
- **Facebook: Jerica Church (just add me as a friend ;)**
- **Text/Call: 801.600.6001**
- **Website: www.selfworthisworthit.com**
- **SCAN QR CODE to Connect - All Things Holistic**

SCAN ME

"A night of peaceful slumber

Unveils a Brighter Dawn."

Chapter 6:

The Magic of Sleep

By Michael Vanderplas

On October 14th, 2012, the Austrian daredevil Felix Baumgartner ascended in a helium balloon capsule to the staggering height of 24 miles above the earth. He had one goal in mind, to break the Guinness Book of World Records for the highest free-fall skydive ever. With his helmet, full body pressure suit, and oxygen tanks all on board, he opened the door to the capsule, stepped outside, and started his ten-minute dive toward the earth below.

Reaching a top speed of 843.6 miles per hour, he broke the sound barrier...WITH HIS BODY!

At one point in time, the pressure related to the speed made him pass out for a short period of time... AS HE WAS ROCKETING TOWARDS THE EARTH!

He regained consciousness, pulled his ripcord, and descended to a soft, controlled touch-down. He did it! Yes, his life was in danger during the skydive, but he broke the world record!

But what does this have to do with sleep?

Well, The Guinness Book of World Records accepted Felix's result by awarding him the world record. However, in 1986 Guinness officially stopped monitoring world records related to sleep deprivation due to the huge negative physical, mental, and emotional hazards related to avoiding sleep.

More than 50 million Americans suffer from some form of sleep deprivation. Chances are that you are one of them. According to recent research from Berkeley University, "Sleep Problems constitute a global epidemic that threatens the health and quality of life for up to 45% of the world's population."

In short, a lack of sleep will impact just about EVERY major physiological aspect of your body and EVERY single operation of your mind. We know this because twice every year, there is a big experiment in which 1.7 billion people across 70 countries take part. We call it daylight savings time and it happens during spring and fall.

Scientists and medical professionals have found that in the spring, when we lose one hour of sleep, there is a 24%

increase in heart attacks the following day. Subsequently, in the fall, when we get an extra hour of sleep (my favorite night of the year), there is a 21% decrease in the number of heart attacks the following day.

If I were to limit your sleep to only 4 hours on only ONE night, there would be almost a 70% decrease in natural killer T-cells activity. Those are the cells that help you kill cancer and fight off disease). Inadequate sleep also has been tied to an increased chance of Alzheimer's, obesity, diabetes, stroke, kidney disease, decreased testosterone levels in men, decreased androgen levels in females, and many more problems.

But it's just not the body. Being a best-selling author on suicide awareness and prevention, I have read dozens of research papers that tie the lack of sleep to increased rates of depression, anxiety, and suicide. The lack of sleep affects every single aspect of our lives and the lives of those we love.

About three years ago, I personally took a deep look into figuring out and focusing on the one thing that would make the biggest difference in my life. What would give me augmented mental clarity, better physical health, enhanced spirituality, and greater emotional resilience? The answer? Sleep.

What Defines "A Good Night's Sleep"?

According to neuroscientist and bestselling author of "Why We Sleep" Mathew Walker, humans need 6-9 hours of continuous sleep daily to not only obtain all the benefits of sleep but also to avoid difficulties related to inadequate sleep. Reportedly, anything less than 6 hours is inadequate.

Like many of us in Western civilization, I used to pride myself in how little sleep I could get and still function. There seems to be a disdain for rest and relaxation in Western civilizations. It's as if we feel like we are being weak to rest and sleep and that our life should be "all about the hustle." In truth, when we round the number of people that are able to sleep less than 6 hours a day on a regular basis and still not suffer any mental, emotional, or physical deficit the next day to the nearest whole number, it is 0 (zero). Zero percent of people are able to function with a deficit. Furthermore, why would you want to sleep less than what is needed?

I could go on for pages and pages more doomsday-ing the horrors of sleeping less than 6-9 hours a night, as well as talk about some of the benefits of a good night's sleep, but I think you get the point. I live by the belief that whenever I see or speak about a problem, it is imperative that I also lay out solutions. Here we go, so get your pen or highlighter out and start marking.

Sleep Hacks

Twenty years ago, in nursing school, I heard a new terminology, "Sleep Hygiene." Just as we need daily care for our physical body to keep it clean, we need daily habits that increase our ability to sleep deeper and for a longer period of time. Being someone that worked night shifts for decades and also suffered from insomnia, I picked up some of the best science-backed tricks of the trade. Here are a few of them.

Become Enlightened

Many times when it's "bedtime," people state that they are not tired. This is likely due to the person not starting their preparation for sleep early enough. So how early in the day should you start the sleep process? Right after you wake up.

You see, in order for us to feel tired, we need to essentially hit our brain's limit of a building block called adenosine. To create adenosine, we need to collect sunlight through the neurotrophin ganglion cells of our eyes. Every cell in our body needs information about the time of the day in order to run our circadian rhythm. When we get out in the sun, the quality and quantity of light absorbed by our eyes is many times greater than by simply using lights in our house, even on cloudy days. This does two things for us. It triggers a release of cortisol to wake us up, and also it sets a timer for the build-up of adenosine which will thus produce the proper levels of melatonin needed for sleep.

Getting outside for 2-10 minutes early in our day without sunglasses is going to be very beneficial. This early light exposure also triggers dopamine release, which gets you motivated to get things done during the day.

In addition, it is important that you avoid bright lights for 90-180 minutes prior to going to bed. This includes the blue light from TVs, computers, and cell phones. Blue light is good during the morning and day but not at night. Early sunlight in the morning and avoiding bright overhead lights at night is the single most important thing you can do to improve your sleep.

Even before getting out of bed, there is another crazy important rule to follow. Avoid the snooze button. Yeah, yeah, I know you've heard this before; however, you probably never heard why. It's called an interruption of sleep inertia.

A normal sleep cycle usually lasts 75-90 minutes. When the alarm wakes you up, you're awake. Yet when you hit that snooze button, you have started another sleep cycle for another 9 minutes until the alarm rings again. That groggy, exhausted feeling is then amplified for the next 4 hours. That makes you less alert, less motivated, and feeling like crap, and can actually lead you down the road to anxiety and depression. Do yourself a favor. Avoid the snooze and embrace your morning superpowers.

Chill Out

Recent studies have found that by decreasing our core body temperature by merely 0.72 degrees Fahrenheit, we are able to increase deep non-REM sleep by 10-20%. In the labs, they have specialized suits that help to decrease the temp at various temperatures. However, you can do this simply by turning your thermostat down a little at night, turning on a fan in the room, or even just putting a cool rag on your head. Many people prefer taking a nice warm shower which raises the body's temperature, and then getting into bed where it will actually cool between 2-4 degrees on average.

The Body Controls the Mind; The Mind Controls the Body.

Has your mind ever been so full that it won't shut off? The problem with that is you spend more brain power focusing on how not to focus. It's a vicious circle of the brain trying not to worry the brain. However, there are simple things we can do with and to our body's senses that help to turn off all the brain's noise.

Focus and slow down on your breathing. When we specifically focus on a longer exhale, our heart rate decreases. This physiological change in the body guides the brain to calm itself. We can slow down our brain even more when we engage in a practice known as Yoga Nidra.

Yoga Nidra is usually done in the savasana pose (lying flat on your back, arms at your sides with your palms facing up). We then focus on our mental awareness of each individual part of the body, or a word presented by the person leading the Yoga Nidra session. It gives your brain something different to focus on instead of the worries of the day. There are a ton of resources out there for you, but I simply look up sessions via YouTube.

Don't underestimate the power of a good sleeping mask or eye shield. I first started using these on long international flights to speaking engagements. They would hand them out in the business section of the plane. I quickly adopted this into my daily life. What the sleeping masks do is close out even more light rays that filter through our eyelids. The darker it is, the better we sleep.

In Closing,

Other aspects not covered in this article to help you sleep are covered in greater detail in my on my YouTube Channel, trainings (reach out to me for details), and my upcoming book on anxiety, available on Amazon.

- How to fall back asleep after waking up at night.
- Lucid Dreaming.
- Calming the Hearing Brain.
- Eye Exhaustion.
- Nutritional Supplements.
- Foods and eating times to enhance quality sleep.
- Light Placement.
- Dream Interpretation.
- Hyper-enhanced Learning via Sleep and Rest.
- Deeper connection with loved ones through Sleep.
- Self-Hypnosis and Sleep.
- Sleep Hacks for night shift workers.
- Sleep Hacks for Travel (short and long distances)

Simply put, what was old is new again. Only now do we have the scientific proof to support what our mothers, grandparents, and ancient ancestors already knew. By adopting both generational and scientific tips, we can unleash the magical powers of sleep in our own lives and add incredible quality to our waking hours.

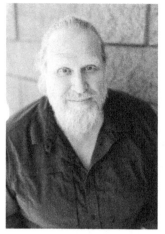

About the Author:
Michael Vanderplas

Michael is a complete healer. As an ICU and Psychiatric Nurse for over 2 decades, Michael has been in more life-and-death situations than most. This has given him incredible insight into the total life spectrum.

Having flown over 1,000,000 miles, his coaching, public speaking, and trainings have taken him to Brazil, Guatemala, El Salvador, Mexico, Canada, Holland, and Australia.

In a lifelong quest to improve himself and those around him, he completed a long-time goal in 2017 to become a Certified Master Trainer of Hypnosis, NLP (Neuro Linguistics Programing), and Quantum TimeLine Therapy.

In 2022 he became an International best-selling author with his debut book "Stay Strong - Overcome Suicidal Thoughts and Live the Life You Always Wanted."
Michael currently works on a daily basis with active-duty military service members, helping them overcome past and present traumas, build resilience, and form healthy relationships with others.

He provides life-changing breakthrough coaching sessions utilizing the most advanced unconscious mind mapping assessment tools on the market. He also provides training certifications in Hypnosis, NLP, and Quantum Timeline Therapy.

 **SCAN QR Code:**

enlightened-academy.com/

YouTube: **Viking** **nurse** @vikingnurse4319

Instagram: mike_vanderplas

facebook.com/Michael.Vanderplas.NLP

"Illuminate Your Mood With
The Brilliance of Light."

Chapter 7:

Shine Your Mental Health
Into Balance With Light

By Marta Lisa Deberard

ave you ever heard that 11:11 is a symbol of intuitive guidance? I believe it after my family received life-changing information about light and its therapeutic power to affect positive physical and emotional change on 11-11-2011.

That was the day we learned that my 75-year-old father was suffering from a dangerous blood clot and wound on his leg. Desperate to add some proactive natural solutions to his wellness routine in order to support a full recovery, my mother remembered the information a trusted friend told us about how shining pads of red, blue, and near-infrared light into the body could increase circulation, prevent infection, and help the body relax into a state of healing. My father began using harmonic light therapy pads at home and could feel an immediate, tingling shift in his sensation. The pulsing light helped his body quickly reduce the swelling, heal the wound, and restore sensation, strength, and mobility to his legs. Applying light to his body didn't just improve the health of his leg; his mental outlook also took a turn away from depression toward optimism.

My mother was so impressed with his results that she started using light therapy. She awoke pain-free each morning for the first time in years, and her overall mood also shifted from anxious worry to peaceful hope. Excited by what I observed in my parents, I tried a 20-minute session with pads of light resting over my closed eyes, mid-back, and belly and experienced a deep feeling of peace and calm. I felt my internal body clock recalibrate, and I was able to wake up feeling refreshed moments before my alarm went off. Excited by these results, I started using light therapy daily and steadily became a more positive, focused, pain-free, and joy-filled person.

I gave light therapy sessions to my friends and yoga students and saw similar amazing results. Applying light physically to the body consistently helped people feel full of light emotionally. The more benefits I experienced and witnessed, the more I wanted to learn how light works. I researched hundreds of clinical studies, consulted with many of the world's leading authorities at conferences, and trained to become a certified light energy coach, product innovator, and educator for a leading light therapy company. My inspired intention is to have people understand and use this powerful modality to shift their physical, mental, emotional, and spiritual health toward optimum vitality.

At our very essence, it is important to remember that we are light beings. Our innate healing capacity is wired to receive light. We are more like plants than we realize; we require light to fuel our minds, body, and spirit. All life turns toward the light, but with our modern lifestyles, most of us spend most of our days inside, blocking the sun, and we seem to have forgotten the wisdom that life requires light. When we don't receive enough of the right light at the right time, it can create physical and emotional imbalances that lead to symptoms of pain, fear, anxiety, and depression. Just notice how you feel different on a bright day of sunshine as opposed to a dark, cloudy day. Scientists today recognize that beyond seasonal affective disorders, light therapy can also help benefit mental health disorders, neurodegeneration, and trauma recovery. Receiving healthy amounts of light can beam us toward balance, help us become more resilient to stress, and help us experience joy, peace, and calm.

In order to shine with light, we need to receive light. We receive most of our light information through our eyes. The eyes are like catcher's mitts for light, and a single particle of light hitting the back of the mitt, the retina, can light up the entire brain. Open or closed, our eyes can send light through the retinal pathway to the hypothalamus and the pineal gland, our third eye in the center of the head, to synchronize us with our natural world and impact our sleep cycles, mood, hormones, intuition, memory, creativity, and consciousness. Through the hypothalamus, light impacts the production of neurohormones to enhance and regulate our mood. Pulsation of this light can also powerfully signal our nervous system to alarm us into fight or flight or calm us into resting, digesting, and healing. Receiving harmonic light can open nervous system pathways that help us move into a state of relaxation and shift our neurohormone production, our circulation, and our gene expression away from stress and inflammation and toward cell preservation and meditative healing.

We also receive light through the skin. Light-sensitive molecules in the energy centers and mitochondria cells throughout our body use visible and near-visible light to increase cellular energy (ATP - Adenosine triphosphate), respiration, and circulation to promote healthy cell function and regeneration. Red and near-infrared light offer the deepest penetration of these benefits into the brain and hard tissue in the body. Blue and green wavelengths help balance liver health and enhance mineral ion exchange. Blue, violet, and ultraviolet wavelengths help the body produce vitamin D and protect it from pathogens. Still, these shorter UV wavelengths can also cause the cellular damage we see with sunburns and skin cancer. Protection from this damage has led us to a lifestyle of hiding from the sun, but we are realizing that we have gone too far and have been reducing healthy light exposure as well.

How do we receive optimal amounts of this critical range of healthy light through our eyes and skin? Visually taking in natural sunlight in the hour around sunrise and sunset is a great place to start. Try to go outside without a hat or sunglasses for twenty minutes daily. Work into your visual exposure slowly if you are light sensitive and do not stare at the sun to receive its benefits. It is helpful to give your skin some direct light exposure in the sun each day before 10:30 am or after 3 pm when the risk of damage from UV light exposure is significantly lower. When indoors, spend daytime hours by windows and natural light as much as possible. At night, sleep in total darkness and away from screens and Wi-Fi devices so that your brain's light-sensitive pineal gland can rest, restore, and signal the release of the sleep neurotransmitter melatonin.

In addition to natural light exposure, supplementing with harmonic light therapy can offer year-round consistent benefits. Different wavelengths of light can offer targeted benefits to the mind and body. Blue-green wavelengths of 465 nm can help boost immunity, calm the nervous system, reset circadian rhythm, and assist with elevated mood and alertness, especially when used in the morning or early afternoon. Amber, Red, and Near-Infrared light wavelengths of 560-880 nm help to increase circulation and cell regeneration which can improve depression, cognition, and brain injury recovery.

To support optimal mental health, I like to use a blue/red or red/infrared light mask over closed eyes for a meditative 20-minute session. To increase the benefit, I add pads of near-infrared light blended with red, blue, or green wavelengths on the belly, and adrenal glands just above the lumbar spine. Light gives the adrenals, which are often taxed in times of long-term mental stress, a chance to recharge and rebalance. Research has shown that light on the gut can improve microbiome diversity, nutrient delivery, and waste elimination. A healthy gut has been directly linked to brain and mood health, as the gut is now known to be critical for the optimal production of neurohormones.

We have used similar harmonic light therapy with thousands of people with impressive results, 94% reported feeling more relaxed, 52% reported feeling lighter, 30% felt happier, and 25% felt more energized after only one session. The Therapeutic Learning Center of Utah gave 586 patients one session a week for four weeks and found that in that month period, 220 patients were able to discontinue their antidepressant medication while under direct supervision. The center found that the light therapy sessions "gave us the ability to work with individual patients and multiple health imbalances with unprecedented ease, speed, and precision."

While a few consistent sessions consistently create a noticeable shift, light therapy's most powerful and lasting effects typically come from regular use. This is why having a light system at home can be so effective. For Alysia Humphries, this has certainly been the case. She writes, "I tried the lights for the first time after we moved to Idaho. Winter was coming, and I was nervous that along with the dark and cold days would come tiredness, lack of motivation, blues, and depression like I had experienced every year, even in sunny Texas. When I tried the lights, I felt energized, peaceful, and more alive. I decided to rent them to try for a few weeks, and I kept feeling better. My kids loved them too. I felt like it was an answer to prayer, and I have continued to use the lights every day to help me stay healthy emotionally and physically. It makes sense to me that light is an important element and nutrient in our health, and just like clean water, and good food, one that is difficult to get enough of nowadays."

When you are looking for ways to improve your health, remember that you are made of light. Healthy light exposure is critical to support your mind and body's ability to heal, regenerate, find balance, and thrive. Keep shining and listening to intuitive nudges; the world needs your LIGHT.

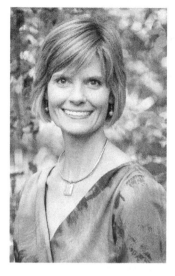

About the Author:
Marta Lisa Deberard

Marta loves being known as the "Light Lady."

Marta is a board-certified Quantum Light Energy Coach who has a passion for educating people about science-based and intuitively effective ways that light nourishes and informs our body, mind, and spirit.

She was an Academic All-American and 4-year varsity volleyball player at the University of North Carolina at Chapel Hill.

Marta has worked for more than 30 years in fitness, yoga, and nutrition education. She began focusing on the exploration and use of light therapy after her family experienced remarkable health results in 2011. Marta holds several patents for innovative harmonic light therapy products and is the lead educator for LumiCeuticals.

SCAN QR Code - You can learn more about the products that Marta works with at lumiceuticals.com, and you can follow posts of information and

research studies and tune into her weekly zoom classes that help empower people toward optimal living at facebook.com/shinewithlight and @shinewithlumi. You can contact her directly at marta@shinewithlight.com

"Sound Healing:

Harmonizing Vibrations, Soothing the Spirit."

Chapter 8:

Sound Healing:
Tune In to Wellness
By Jhill Seraphina

I've always been drawn to healing, nurturing, and taking care of people. I started out as a massage therapist, happy to provide relaxation and physical relief to my clients. Ten years into my massage career, I felt called to energy work to further help my clients on their healing journey.

After getting attuned to the highest level in the Japanese healing modality of Reiki, there was a little bit of a struggle incorporating energy work into my practice. Massage therapy is very physical, hands-on, and practical, whereas Reiki is more energetic, intuitive, and hands-off. I eventually found my groove with it, and clients were loving the deeper level of healing they were experiencing in their sessions.

Around this same time, I had my first exposure to sound healing. At the end of a yoga session, the instructor walked around with a crystal singing bowl, and it pierced my soul, unlike anything I had ever felt before! It felt like seeing the sun for the first time after a long winter; like a cold drink of water in the middle of the desert. My body wanted more, and I immediately knew I needed this in my life! I ordered a crystal bowl and started intuitively adding it to my clients' sessions, and they loved it!

I then sought out training and got certified as a sound healing practitioner and have seen countless miracles in myself, my friends, my family, and clients with vibrational medicine. I love that sound healing covers the full spectrum; it's practical, physical, and hands-on like massage, and yet also intuitive and energetic like Reiki. This was the missing key for me, and I am now so passionate about the healing powers of vibrational medicine.

In recent years, sound healing has become an increasingly popular form of therapy for individuals looking to boost their mental health. Sound healing is a holistic therapy that uses sound vibrations to promote physical, emotional, and mental well-being. Practice can involve using different types of instruments, such as singing bowls, gongs, tuning forks, and even your voice, to produce vibrations that help relax the mind and body and resonate at their proper levels.

The reason sound healing works so well on our bodies is because of two scientific terms: entrainment and sympathetic resonance. Entrainment is when two objects that are in a similar motion yet at different rates will sync up to be in motion together just by being near each other. This phenomenon can be observed in a flock of birds all flapping their wings in coordination and also with pendulum-hanging clocks on a wall. If all the pendulums are swinging at different rates, within an hour, they will be moving in precise motion with each other. This is because nature seeks the most efficient functional state. It takes less energy to pulse in cooperation than in opposition.

The term sympathetic resonance comes from the idea that one object is sympathetic to the vibrations of another object and begins to vibrate in response, even without being directly struck. For example, when someone laughs out loud near my gong, it will start to sing. When I'm drumming on the floor, the chimes hanging from the ceiling can start to play their harmonic tones. Objects that were previously not in motion become in motion due to exposure to nearby vibrations. Entrainment and sympathetic resonance can be used to restore harmonious body functions, which are both at work in sound healing treatments.

When parts of our body are out of balance, we can retune them, similar to tuning a piano. If a piano is out of tune, do we get mad and rip out the insides? No, we simply tune it back up! We must take the same approach for our bodies rather than turning to surgeries and medicines as the first step.

"There will come a time when a diseased condition will not be described as it is today by physicians and psychologists, but it will be spoken of in musical terms, as one would speak of a piano that was out of tune."– Rudolph Steiner

Each organism has its own vibratory rate. Every object in the universe has its own unique resonant frequency. Resonance can be demonstrated when one tuning fork is struck and placed next to another tuning fork. The second fork begins to resonate with the first fork, and sound waves from the first tuning fork impart their energy to the second one. When an opera singer shatters a glass with her voice, they match the resonant frequency of the glass and set it into vibration. Our bodies can also resonate with the frequency of sound, and during a sound healing session, your body gets to come into alignment with healing vibrations.

Sound can travel 760 miles per hour in the air, but 3,350 miles per hour in water. The human body is composed of 70% water, which makes it a very good conductor of sound. Every organ, bone, and cell in our body has its individual frequency, and when they work together, they create frequencies similar to instruments in an orchestra. If one organ or instrument is out of tune, it affects the whole body.

Every day, we are exposed to frequencies that can be negative and harmful, and if a person feels physically or mentally ill, several of their body functions might be working out of harmony. A sound healer can produce strong, clear, harmonious vibrations, plus healing intent, and their body will lock into the powerful healing frequency where harmony is restored, often avoiding the need for medical intervention.

The beauty of sound healing is that words don't need to be spoken in order for healing to occur. Clients don't have to divulge vulnerable details or relive traumatic experiences. The vibrations are able to identify, pull up, and shift any stagnant or low frequencies in our body naturally and gently. Sound healing instruments, like Tibetan metal bowls, crystal singing bowls, shamanic drums, and gongs are powerful in their ability to help process emotions.

Tuning forks can be used for instantly shifting and improving vibrations. They are convenient to keep in purses, bags, bedside tables, and even in cars. Tuning forks come in two options: weighted or unweighted. Weighted forks have round weights at the end of each prong and work by placing the stem directly on the body, once activated. They don't make much sound as the vibrations travel down through the stem and right into your body. Unweighted forks are sleeker as they don't have the weights on the end. These are held a few inches above the body and make an audible sound as the vibrations travel up and out through the prongs.

For example, every morning, I strike two unweighted tuning forks together and hold them near my ears and point them at my heart when I wake up. I do this for two minutes in an effort to charge my energetic field and set my intentions for the day. If I ever need a shift in my mood or feel anxious and need to feel more grounded, I love to use a weighted tuning fork on my feet and instantly feel more balanced and calmer.

Sound healing is an effective form of healing because our bodies are made of energy. Therefore, it has vibrations, and vibrations are easily influenced to change. The vibrations of our bodies are affected by a myriad of lifestyle choices: the foods we eat, the thoughts we think, the environments we are exposed to, etc. But sometimes, our vibrations are lowered by things out of our control, such as depression, addiction, anxiety, bacteria/viruses, etc. Hence, we need to be aware and intentional about our energetic health.

Just like we can take vitamins to help supplement our nutrient intake and boost our body's ability to function properly, we can also purposefully add healing vibrations to our energetic field and raise our vibrations so that we can experience peak performance and optimal health.

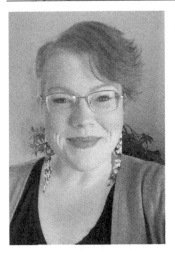

About the Author:
Jhill Seraphina

Jhill Seraphina is an intuitive holistic healer with a passion for helping people live their best life. She loves helping clients escape feeling stuck, overwhelmed, burned out, and any other kind of emotional trauma.

Whether she's providing individualized care in her office or doing sound baths at festivals, conferences, and retreats, Jhill makes everyone feel brighter, lighter, and happier!

Jhill's studio, Vibes of Light, is located in Salt Lake City, where she is available for in-person appointments, sound baths, and workshops.

Jhill offers training and certifications for sound healing as well as Reiki. She can do energy sessions over the phone and has clients all over the US. She believes that the key to achieving true health and wellness is to address the root cause of any imbalances in the body, rather than simply treating the symptoms, therefore working the mind, body, and spirit in every session.

Trained / Licensed / Certified

- Massage Therapy

- Sound Healing
- Reiki Master
- Shamanism of the Andean Lineage
- Craniosacral Therapy
- Light Therapy
- Essential Oils
- Muscle Testing
- Ho'oponopono
- Breathwork
- Bachelor's Degree in Business Administration from Southern New Hampshire University

You can learn more about the services Jhill offers with Vibes of Light at:

 **QR Code to:**
www.VibesofLightHealing.com
www.instagram.com/vibesoflight
www.facebook.com/jhillseraphina
You can contact her directly at
jhillseraphina@gmail.com

"Crystals:

Earth's whispers, nurturing with gentle energy."

Chapter 9:

Crystal Energy

By Sara Anderson

Many years ago, a friend asked if I happened to have some specific stones and crystals. At the time, I was working as a nurse, but had access to a rock business. I asked her what she wanted them for and she told me that she was using them for their healing properties, and that when she held them, she could feel them vibrate in her hand. What?! I told her she was crazy!

My journey into the alternative healing world began in 2011. At that time, I had been in the medical field for about ten years. After a lifetime of fighting a diagnosis of IBS (Irritable Bowel Syndrome), I was scheduled for major surgery. The medical field's only answer was surgery.

I wasn't ready to put my body through that, so I searched for an alternative answer. My aunt had introduced me to an iridologist years before, so I thought maybe she could give me a healthier direction. (Iridology is the study of the patterns in the eyes to determine any physical ailments that may be present in the body. This practitioner gave me a long list of supplements needed to support healthier body function but then she said, "Energy work would change all this."

Well, of course, I was intrigued! And boy did it change my life!

This amazing world of recognizing and healing stuck emotions and healing generational trauma was an eye-opener to a whole new world! My body had an immediate result from the very first visit! I had such a miraculous result that I never had the surgery, never went back to a doctor, and after about a year, my body started to function properly on its own. Mind-blowing right?! My nurse's brain wanted to know what the heck had just happened! So, I signed up for classes, and let me tell you, it took years for my nurse brain to wrap around this new concept. My biggest "aha" was how emotions have a direct effect on the body. I had been good at holding in all my emotions all my life. And as a nurse, I liked to "take pain away" from my patients.

In my studies, I found multiple tools along my way...essential oils, emotional release, tapping, reiki, foot zoning, chakra balancing, herbs, and supplements, and yes, eventually, I discovered crystal energy.

I started to really focus on the energy of stones and how they affected the body's energy field. After a couple years of being a "traveling rock shop", I was inspired to open a physical location. On January 28, 2020, I opened doors to The Crystal Corner (great year to open a business!), in my hometown. I wanted to create a space for people to gather and enjoy the beautiful creations of the earth while feeling peace, unity, and unconditional love. At The Crystal Corner, we aim to feed your soul with love and acceptance, so that when you come in, you can experience a little break from the crazy chaos in the world. We are a community space of hope and healing, disguised as a rock shop.

Crystal Energy:

"Everything is energy, and that's all there is to it. This is not philosophy. This is physics." -Albert Einstein.

Science has proven that most matter is empty space, and what makes up this empty space is energy. Energy is everything, and everything is energy. You, your phone, the chair you are sitting on, and the crystals in your pocket are all vibrating energy. As a human, your vibration is unstable and easily influenced. It constantly changes as we are exposed to other people, the news, family, the weather, and even our own memories. Crystals, on the other hand, have a stable energy frequency that doesn't change. They have fixed, permanent, geometric shapes that maintain that perfect stability without any effort. Why does that matter? Well, more stable energy equals more powerful energy, and powerful energies influence the energies around it.

Every crystal has a different energetic frequency. The influences on the crystal can include the size, the composition, and, most important is, the color. Why is color so important? Well, the colors we see are actually light frequencies. Think about a rainbow. A rainbow is caused when light enters a water droplet, slowing down and bending. Sunlight is made up of many wavelengths or colors of light. Some of those wavelengths get bent more than others. So, the shortest wavelength (violet) bends the most, and red bends the least, so the colors are always in the same order...violet, indigo, blue, green, yellow, orange, and red. Do you know the chakra colors? They are in the exact same order from head to toe! The shorter the wavelength, the higher the frequency. For example, the color violet has a short wavelength and shows up as the highest frequency in the crown chakra.

Because of the vibrational match with colors, you can usually choose your crystal by matching the chakra you want to balance. (If you don't remember about chakras, review Chapter 5 in this book went more in-depth about chakras). And if you are not sure what chakra you want to work on, just pick the crystal that your intuition guides you to! Your own body intuitively knows what it needs, so lean into trust. My favorite is when a customer comes in that knows nothing about crystal healing, and I suggest they just choose what stands out to them. After they let go of judgment, get out of their head, and step into their body, we talk about the stone they choose. Most are blown away by what I can tell them about their body or life situation by the stone they choose! I don't proclaim to be a psychic; I just understand how the various stones affect us!

Some stones have physical energy that can be seen more easily. My favorite stone of all is called Genesis Stone.

It is a combination of magnetite, hematite, and jasper and can be dated to be over a billion years old! Its structure has magnetic properties, so a magnet sticks to it. This magnetic property, when placed on the body, promotes increased blood flow, which may decrease inflammation, which then aids migraines, headaches, arthritis, backaches, and all kinds of pain issues. Many of my friends and customers have the Genesis Stone on their vehicle seats to aid in back pain while driving! It also may align with water molecules when placed in your drinking water to create "structured water", which the body absorbs more efficiently. Another example of a common stone used in water is shungite, which is a carbon, and carbons are known to be used in water filters to detoxify the water we drink. So many of you already drink what my kids call "rock water"! Haha!

Crystals work best when you don't just leave them to do all the work themselves. For best results, pair the crystal's natural energy with your own clear thoughts and intentions. It's proven that where your thoughts go, energy flows. So, use your crystals to amplify your positive thoughts and intentions. Some think crystal energy is just a placebo effect. While it can get a bad rap, the placebo effect is real and strongly supported by research.

The power of positive thought has been shown to affect health outcomes in patients undergoing treatments. And, like anything related to health and wellness, from juicing to meditation, crystals can be an addition to your healing journey, but I never advise it to be a substitute for working with your trusted medical professional. Our well-being can't all be summed up by numbers and data, but if crystals can

support us in a way that we can't see, but we can *feel*, isn't that powerful enough?

About the Author:
Sara Anderson

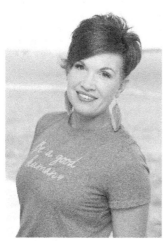

Sara is the owner and creator of The Crystal Corner, a retail space located in Tremonton Utah. She has been in the medical field for over 20 years as a Licensed Practical Nurse (LPN). At a young age, Sara knew her purpose in life would be to help people in their healing journey.

Sara's passion for bringing hope and healing to her community has created a retail space with crystals, jewelry, and home decor, paired with a Zen Den Yoga Studio that hosts several informational, metaphysical, and spiritual events. The store offers a variety of classes, including wire wrapping, science behind crystal grids, chakra balancing, new and full moon energy, and free teen club and adult resiliency support group.

Sara is certified in BioEnergetic Synchronization Technique (B.E.S.T). This technique is a gentle healing system that addresses the whole being and promotes balance in the body.

Sara believes we have compassion for each other when we first have compassion for ourselves. May Light and Love lead your way every day.

SCAN QR Code to:
CrystalCornerShop.com

https://www.facebook.com/Thecrystalcornerutah

https://www.instagram.com/thecrystalcornerutah/

"Meditation:

Unveiling the power within, beyond the noise."

Chapter 10:

Power through Meditation

By Kristi Corless

Over 14 years ago before I ever knew about foot zoning, essential oils, or any alternative health modalities, I found myself lying on the floor at an event with other people, "meditating" I don't remember if it was a guided meditation, or if we were just lying there allowing whatever inspiration needed to come to us, but what I do remember is it changed my life forever.

At the time, I was trying to conceive my son. I had struggled with infertility (endometriosis) and adopted my first two children 3 and a half years apart.

I knew this next one was to come through me, so I was in constant prayer and searching for answers.

As I lay on that floor that day, I was asking if I could catch a glimpse of my future baby. Some friends had mentioned seeing dreams or visions of their children before having them, and I felt like it was an ok thing to seek. So, I laid there breathing in, trying to clear my mind...and I had a rush of images and events flood my mind and thoughts. I did catch a glimpse of my son. And so much more!

I came home and wrote down everything I could remember in my journal. I was in awe.

The next weeks, months, and years passed, and I conceived and gave birth to my son. His eyes are like the ones I saw in that meditation. The older he gets the more familiar they are.

I meditated here and there, mostly on my own, and took time to quiet my mind and gather answers to questions, kind of like an extension of prayer. I started my foot zoning training, and went on to learn back zoning, face zoning, and hand zoning. I was teaching essential oil classes and at this time I had started praying for the "gift of discernment" At the end of this Emotions and essential oils class I was teaching, I talked with this lady, and I could tell she had the ability to discern, and she was using it to help people with their healing. I expressed my desire and that I had been praying for this. She turned to me and looked me directly in the eyes and said," You have that gift, the angels are all around, and they are telling me you just need to be quiet and listen."

It was like all the lights came on for me that day, not just a single bulb over my head. All the lights turned on, like a thousand suns shining all at once!

I took more time to be still and listen. That's as simple as meditation needs to be. Get off our electronic devices, walk away from the distractions and stresses of life, be still, and listen.

I learned when I was stressed, I could take some deep breaths and be still, even though there were storms of chaos around me. I could meditate, I could listen to my inner calm. As I felt happier, more connected, and clearer, I started getting interested in how this was helping the brain scientifically.

I found out that meditation helps reduce cytokines, which are the inflammatory stress chemicals that can lead to depression. It also calms anxiety and racing thoughts. It can boost self-confidence, as we can feel more in control and empowered in every situation. You see meditation isn't just lying on the floor or sitting in the lotus position saying "ohmm." It's pausing, taking a few deep breaths to reset, stopping the typical freak-out response. Coming back to our true powerful center, to respond in a different way than past programming would respond. It's interrupting that former neural pathway and creating a healthier one.

I enjoy longer meditations too. With life and busy schedules, I recommend if you don't already meditate, start with just 3 minutes. You could even set a timer.

Put on an instrumental hymn or classical piece if you'd like. I do feel music enhances my meditation. Start with a question or something you want to let go of, or a need you would like support or guidance with. or a one-word intention like "peace" "love" "forgive" "joy" or "abundance."

Next, choose a consistent time to meditate. Morning is a great time to set intentions for the day and visualize how you'd like your day to go. Yet, for you night owls, evening can also be a powerful time to meditate and to set intentions for the next day.

There are no wrong ways to meditate. Well, I guess if you had the tv on, earbuds blasting a loud song and teenagers or toddlers talking to you all at once...that could not be ideal for meditation, haha. Meditation is more of an art, so have fun with it. Try it at different times of day, with different music in the background. See what works best for you to stay consistent.

Really, it can be easy. You can start by taking a few deep breaths, releasing any stresses, doubts, worries, fears, darkness, and heaviness... let it all go with each exhale, give yourself permission to breathe it out...let it go... surrender. With every inhale, breathe in the love, peace, light, and joy that surrounds you.

I believe in angels, so I will tell you, if that's your belief as well, to listen to whispers from them. Have a pen and paper close to write down thoughts and ideas that they share, or that come to your heart and mind. It's nice to look back and see your insights and answers.

97

Remember my journal? I had written down my insights from that first meditation fourteen years ago. Well, four or five years ago I was working with a man who could play the "music of your soul." It helped people release emotions and connect more with themselves, becoming more aware and mindful. I started doing guided meditations with him. We'd have group events, and He'd start playing, and I'd start speaking...the words would flow out of me. For each group, it was exactly what was needed.

I started thinking about creating a CD or download so people could have one anytime, anywhere, to help them. I didn't feel like he was the right fit for the music though. I either remembered this or came across my entry in my journal one day as I was pondering. It said, "Get healing music from Mark Stevenson."

I remembered my friend who worked with him as her arranger, and I had met him one day, and he talked a little about healing frequencies and how powerful they could be, even with cancers! At that time of my meditation, he was the one I was prompted to write down in my journal for the healing music I would need for the future.

When I needed it, I was able to go back and find the information needed to contact him. With his help with healing frequencies and my favorite hymns, he arranged beautiful music in the key and order of the energy centers (chakras) for overall support. I wrote down some thoughts and opened my mouth at his studio in front of his microphone and 52 minutes of a healing guided meditation called Immersed in His Light came to be.

As you meditate, you may see colors or see images or symbols, in your mind's eye or clearly. Others may feel things in their body, and tune into those to connect with and release/heal trapped emotions or energy. Others may get words and thoughts flowing through. Some may experience this and more. Whatever your abilities, strengths, or gifts, they can and will develop and grow stronger as you practice.

My friends, old and new, who may be reading this, please take time to be still, listen, meditate, and write things down. You may be searching for answers. Are you asking and asking, and still feel stuck? The answers are all around you, (inside of you, in your heart, and outside of you). Be still and listen, practice disconnecting from the world and tuning into you and your higher power and angels support around you. You'll know how to take action. Hugs and prayers, Love, and Light to you as you continue on your journey! You've got this!!!

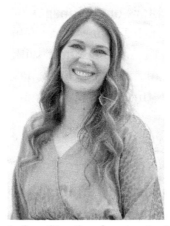

About the Author:
Kristi Corless

Kristi has 4 beautiful children aged 12, 13, 17, and 20.

She has an amazing supportive husband.

She struggled with infertility (endometriosis) and adopted 2 children, 1 came through in vitro and 1 the "old fashioned" way after finding natural answers to her challenges.

Her mission is to help others find natural healing solutions too. She has been sharing and educating through the vehicle of dōTERRA®, with their unparalleled products for over 12 years.

She has 13 years of experience and 10 certifications in alternative healing methods including foot, back, face, and hand zoning, Access bars, Reiki, Bones I, Bones II (deep emotional releasing) the Aroma touch back technique. She's a certified Life coach. She created her own technique called "Instant Release," and the illumination method which is the blueprint for her own certification course "Illumination."

She has an intuitive ability to lead people through guided meditations, visualizations, or conversations & communicate those messages that are exactly what they need to hear to clear physical, mental, emotional, and spiritual blocks, reconnect deeper to their true self and higher power to shine their light brighter than ever before, and live their true purpose with more vision, confidence, and clarity.

She is passionate about assisting others in developing their gifts and reminding them that the answers are all within. "Be still, listen, meditate, then act. We are not alone, always remember your Angels and Higher power are all around to help you! Your success is Inevitable!"

 **SCAN QR CODE: Women's Health Class**

https://vimeo.com/806211101/885f121a3a

"Embrace Wholeness,

Let Pain Dissolve Into Distant Memories."

Chapter 11:

Flipping Your Bioelectrical Switch
Out of Survival Mode

By MarLeice Hyde

I *always knew I wanted to be a nurse. My mom tells the story of me at 5 years old following the nurses around when my grandpa was in the hospital, pretending to check his pulse and listen with the stethoscope. As a teen, my best friend and I started a volunteer program at the local hospital. I studied in after-school programs to certify as a CNA (Certified Nursing Assistant) and as a senior in high school I became Wyoming's youngest EMT. (Emergency Medical Technician).*

I graduated from BYU with my Bachelors in Nursing and gained experience in cardiology, oncology, pediatrics, orthopedics, memory care, addiction recovery, and management in the Salt Lake City region then in the emergency room when I moved to California. I completed a Master's Degree in Nursing Leadership & Education in 2010 and began teaching at nursing school which was my dream job. When the school was sold, I ended up creating a pain clinic at a local doctor's office & became a specialist in CRPS (chronic regional pain syndrome), a.k.a the suicide disease. Why is all this history important? So many years in the mainstream medical field had me very entrenched and brainwashed about how things should be done: standard "protocols" (i.e., chemicals - drugs). Many clients had lost hope, having been told repeatedly by doctors they'd have to "live with it" (the pain), and only option was to swallow pills the rest of their lives.

I was born with a congenital hip defect, missing a proper socket in the bone for the ball of the femur to be stabilized by. I didn't discover this fact until my late 20's however, when my hip completely dislocated for the first time after catching a patient falling which tore all the muscles that had been doing the stabilizing job so well during my athletic youth. It was never the same after that, and every step started stabbing like a knife as I developed a noticeable limp. I was terrified!

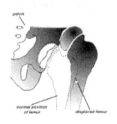

My brother had the same problem, only worse, and I watched what he went through as a teen and young adult, with a rare, difficult surgery on the East Coast to first break his pelvis and then rebuild and replace his hip joint. It took him nearly a year to recover and learn to walk again- I didn't want to go through that. By early 2015 I was becoming desperate, the choice becoming critical to either accept the surgery or live life from a wheelchair. It was at this desperate juncture I was invited to a training seminar in Texas by Dr. John Hache about Microcurrent Biofeedback Neuromodulation Therapy. I learned that every type of cell in the body communicates at its own electrical frequency- like tuning a radio. And that electricity precedes chemistry. When a heart stops, it's not chemicals that get it going again, it's electricity! If we only understood how low voltage affects our health on a cellular level, we would look to frequency and electricity for solutions (as Tesla did) instead of chemicals and recharge our body as often as our phone. I learned that microcurrent algorithms can provide up to 500x more energy than any other modality.

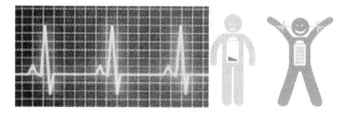

I also began to understand the critical difference with devices (Check out my bio for the microcurrent device I recommend): the body's own electrical language, a biphasic damped sine wave instead of a square wave like traditional TENS and even other "Microcurrent" devices. Which takes millions of measurements per second (biofeedback), changes the signal as needed to respond to the body's communication and prevents adaptation (neuromodulation). This means they COMMUNICATE with the body instead of trying to DOMINATE it or BLOCK nerve signals temporarily. This is critical to understand!

Picture the body having miles of electrical rivers (called fascia) flowing everywhere: blockages (like beaver dams and swamps) are caused by inflammation or scar tissue, resulting in the brain perceiving those blockages (lack of energy) as pain signals. These devices can locate the blockages and use the correct frequencies to heal/remove them permanently. Not simply treating or masking symptoms, actually fixing the problem. This opened my mind to the possibilities for real healing. My personal paradigm completely shifted.

Then Dr. Hache demonstrated a body alignment technique on me, electrically reprogramming the muscle tissue. When I stood up five (only FIVE!) minutes later, I was walking with no pain and no limp. I cried because it felt so good, and it gave me back the HOPE that had been stripped away by traditional medicine. I purchased the technology on the spot, practiced, and became proficient, and opened my own clinic that Fall. I also began teaching seminars with Dr. Hache, and he was my mentor until COVID-19 shut down in-person events.

I learned many things about the nervous system and pain signals while working with my CRPS (Complex regional pain syndrome) clients at this time. Primarily I learned that the nervous system could send severe pain signals with no physical reason in a phenomenon known as "phantom pain." Imagine spraining your ankle. It hurts very badly for a few days, then the pain gets less and disappears as the injury heals. With CRPS, the pain never lessens even when the structure heals, and then it starts to spread to other parts of the body also. This unremitting pain keeps their body in constant stress mode. Many CRPS clients are diagnosed by psychiatrists because doctors don't believe them. Many I worked with waited a decade or more for an accurate diagnosis. The ketamine (Ketamine is a fast-acting anesthetic and painkiller) we infused saturates the glial cells (same receptors as opiates), calming down the panicked nerves and lessening the pain signals but they needed very expensive 4-hour infusions (that insurance didn't cover) every few weeks to maintain the relief after the initial 6-week jumpstart protocol.

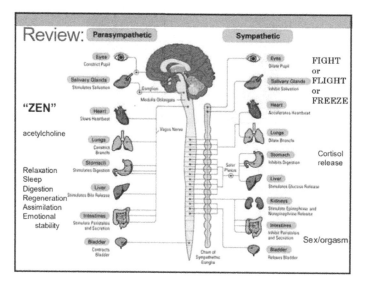

The body has two primary states of being: Stress/Survival mode (aka fight/flight/freeze) and Zen mode. The body exists in one or the other at any given time. Imagine being chased by a wolf... in survival mode, your heart rate speeds up, your hands get cold as blood is shunted to the core organs, your pupils open wide to see better, your mouth goes dry, your blood sugar goes up, cortisol and other endorphins are released, etc. All the other body systems turn off: you don't have to stop and go to the bathroom, you're wide awake, and your stomach clenches. You couldn't possibly eat, sleep, learn, be calm, or heal. When someone is in chronic pain, the body stays in this survival mode which prevents healing. So, the challenge becomes, how do we get the body back into Zen mode?

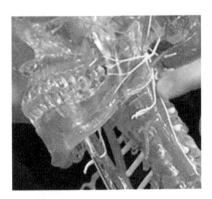

The simple answer is there is a master nerve that flips the switch out of Survival mode back into Zen mode: the Vagus Nerve. One on each side of the body, they are the longest cranial nerves which connect the brainstem to the heart, diaphragm, and gut, branching out to all abdominal organs and terminate in the feet. They are the control center for the parasympathetic nervous system: they regulate inflammation body-wide and also manage and process emotions.

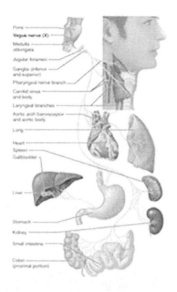

There are many ways to stimulate the Vagus Nerve, which slams the brakes on survival mode. Some easy natural ways include humming or "OHM-ing", mantra-chanting, Hymn singing, especially in a group, MILD exercise, half-smile position (and other Yoga & Tai Chi maneuvers), splashing your face with cold water, Valsalva maneuver/bearing down, gargling, Meditation, Affirmations, hugging, healing music, or watching a candle flame.

Some stronger physical ways to activate the Vagus nerve include direct stimulation of the diaphragm by: Diaphragmatic breathing, laughing, and jumping on a trampoline. You can also directly activate it by using two fingers to tap or massage the neck area an inch below the ear behind the SCM muscle (sternocleidomastoid muscle) repeatedly. Do only one side at a time, not both together! This kind of stimulation can pull you out of a panic attack, relieve migraine, and relax muscle spasms.

Of course, the easiest, best, and most effective way to stimulate the Vagus nerve is with direct application of microcurrent therapy in the right place at the right frequency. My CRPS clients and I started experimenting with microcurrent during their treatment sessions. We learned that 6-10 minutes of Direct Vagus Nerve Stimulation (VNS) with microcurrent gave as much or more pain relief than a 4-hour ketamine infusion. Many clients were able to totally stop chemical infusions when they started doing daily VNS with microcurrent at home. Talk about life-changing!

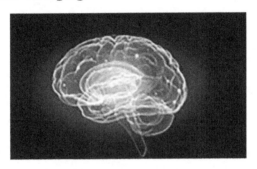

There is one more thing I want to mention: the connection between chronic pain and sleep deprivation. Your brain has five basic frequencies or vibrational states. Zen mode is when the brain is in an Alpha state vibrating between 7-12 Hz, (which encompasses the 7.83 base frequency of the Earth aka the Schumann Resonance). This is where we mostly want to be when we are awake.

Survival mode vibrates in the Beta zone as high as 35 Hz (triple the normal speed)! If you are in Survival mode when it's time to sleep, imagine how long it takes to slow the brain down not only to the alpha state around 8 Hz, but all the way down to 1-4 Hz, where REM sleep happens. The longer you spend in Survival Mode, the more the other body systems shut down and the harder it is to slow the brain down enough to reach REM or dream sleep. When my CRPS clients received their infusions, they were given medication to help them sleep and prevent side effects. At least half the benefit of these infusions was 4 solid hours of REM sleep which many hadn't achieved in years.

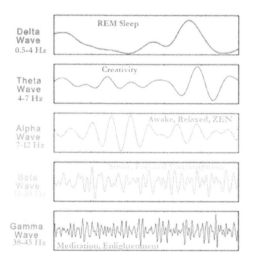

Why is REM sleep so important? During REM sleep, the brain recalibrates, takes out the trash, drops cortisol levels, converts short-term to long-term memory & does general repair & regeneration. If you never reach your dream sleep, none of those activities happen. And the less REM sleep you get the more the pain/stress takes over: a vicious cycle very difficult to break and one key element of chronic pain relief. It can take hours of sleep to reach this dream state so sleep cycles frequently interrupted by pain may never get there. But using Microcurrent therapy to generate the Delta frequency, clients can be assisted into REM sleep which breaks the chronic pain cycle and begins the long-term healing process.

Professional-level Microcurrent Devices generate all 5 brain waves. Gamma waves can help reprogram the brain to alleviate PTSD symptoms. Delta waves not only help people sleep but reprogram the brain to lessen depression. Theta waves stimulate creativity. Beta waves can relieve symptoms of narcolepsy. Finally, of course, Alpha waves do the most effective form of Vagus Nerve Stimulation available and so much more!

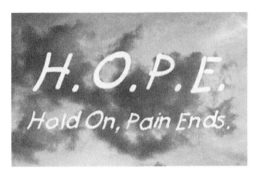

I look forward to connecting with you to assist you in your own journey to go from crazy chaos to calm, to reclaim HOPE.

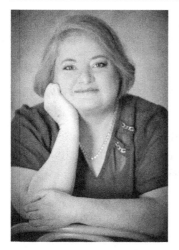

About the Author:
MarLeice Hyde, MSN, RN, CTIH

MarLeice Hyde, MSN, RN, CTIH started her healthcare career as an EMT before graduating high school as one of Wyoming's Presidential Scholars in 1993. She progressed through CNA, LVN, and finally to RN as she graduated from BYU with her BSN.

MarLeice completed her Master's Degree in Nursing Leadership & Education in 2010. She was introduced to AvazziaLife Pinnacle microcurrent therapy in 2015, which markedly improved her own health instantly, so she quickly became a professional practitioner and opened the Erasing Pain Holistic Healing Center in Sacramento, CA.

MarLeice has used her prior electrical stimulation experience to advance the applications of the technology, creating accessories to make therapy easier to administer for both patients and practitioners.

With now more than 30 years of experience encompassing both traditional and alternative medical therapies, she creates connections, acting as a bridge between Eastern and Western philosophies, Allopathic and Holistic traditions. She is currently known as the

113

Microcurrent Missionary: using, distributing, and teaching the miracle of Avazzia and AvazziaLife Microcurrent devices, in particular, the AvazziaLife Pinnacle Device.

MarLeice's goal as a life coach is to empower and assist each client to progress through her 5 Pillars of Erasing Pain (Physical healing, Nutritional support, Detoxification, EMF Protection, and Emotional release) to achieve their own maximum health and happiness.

 **SCAN QR CODE: Erasingpain.com @erasingpain.com You can purchase AvazziaLife Pinnacle Microcurrent devices at** www.shopmicrocurrent.com. **You can be trained on how to use them with pre-recorded classes at** www.learnmicrocurrent.com. **And you can schedule a free 15-minute consultation with me personally at** www.erasingpain.com.

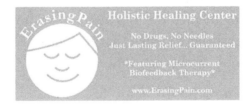

"Let's Create a Home Space
That's Your Happy Place."

Chapter 12:

How Your Home Can Help You
Go From Crazy To Calm

By Kathy Watts

As I stood in the middle of my living room, frantically searching for my phone, I couldn't help but feel frustrated. I had an important call scheduled in just a few minutes and couldn't afford to be late. My husband chuckled as he overheard me mumbling to myself, "Where's my phone?"

It was then that I realized how often I said those words. It had become a reflex for me to panic whenever I couldn't find something I needed. But why was that? Was it just me, or did everyone else feel the same way? Determined to find answers, I started researching. It turns out it's not uncommon for people to feel overwhelmed when they can't locate their belongings. In fact, it can trigger a stress response in the brain and make you feel like you're losing control.

Your home is your sanctuary. It's where you come to relax, unwind, and spend time with the people you love. But sometimes, despite your best efforts, your homes can feel chaotic and cluttered, making it difficult to find what you need.

If you're tired of feeling overwhelmed by your living space, it's time to take action. In this chapter, we'll explore tips to transform your home from a chaotic mess to a peaceful haven. From decluttering tips to aromatherapy, we'll cover everything you need to know to create a calming atmosphere in your living space. Whether you're struggling with a small apartment or a large family home, we've got you covered. So, get ready to say goodbye to stress and hello to Zen vibes in your home.

The Importance of a Peaceful Home

Your home is more than just a place to eat and sleep. It's a reflection of your personality and your lifestyle. A peaceful home can profoundly impact your mental and physical health. When surrounded by clutter and chaos, it can be difficult to relax and unwind. A peaceful home, on the other hand, can help you feel calmer and more centered, making it easier to manage stress and anxiety.

Creating a peaceful home is about more than just aesthetics. It's about creating a space that feels comfortable and inviting, a place where you can truly be yourself. When your home is peaceful, you're more likely to feel energized and motivated, which can positively impact all areas of your life.

Identifying Clutter and Chaos in Your Living Space

The first step in creating a peaceful home is identifying clutter and chaos in your living space. This can be daunting, especially if you've lived in the same place for a long time.

Start by taking a good look around your home. What do you see? Are there piles of books and magazines on the coffee table? Is the kitchen counter covered in appliances and utensils? Are there clothes spilling out of your closet? These are all signs of clutter and chaos.

Take note of the areas of your home that feel overwhelming or stressful. Is it the bedroom, the living room, or the kitchen? Once you've identified the problem areas, you can start taking action to declutter and organize your space.

Sometimes you need additional help to declutter your space. This is why I wrote the Home Compass System. In the Home Compass, you release emotions that could be the root cause of your clutter.

Work through what clutter you can, and if you get stuck and need extra help, contact us! I have the Home Compass workbook on Amazon, plus an 11-week workshop class.

The Benefits of Decluttering

Decluttering your home can be daunting, but the benefits are worth the effort. When you declutter your living space, you create a more peaceful environment that is easier to manage and maintain. Here are just a few of the benefits of decluttering:

- Reduced stress and anxiety
- Increased productivity and focus
- Improved sleep and relaxation
- More space for the things you love
- A more organized and efficient home

Decluttering your home can also have a positive impact on your mental health. When you let go of the things you no longer need or use, you create more space for the things that truly matter. This can help you feel more focused and energized, positively impacting your overall well-being.

Decluttering Tips for Every Room in Your Home

Now that you understand the benefits of decluttering, it's time to start. Here are some decluttering tips for every room in your home:

The Living Room

- Start by removing anything that doesn't belong in the living room, such as dishes or laundry.
- Remove any items that are broken, damaged, or no longer used.
- Donate or sell any items in good condition but no longer needed.
- Store items used less frequently, such as seasonal decorations, in a closet or storage container.

- Use organizers and storage solutions to keep items such as books, magazines, and remote controls tidy and accessible.

The Kitchen

- Start by removing everything from your cabinets and drawers.
- Discard any expired or unused food items.
- Donate or sell any kitchen gadgets or appliances that you no longer use.
- Use organizers and storage solutions to organize pots, pans, and utensils.
- Invest in a few high-quality storage containers for pantry items such as pasta, rice, and cereal.

The Bedroom

- Start by removing everything from your closet and dresser.
- Discard any items that are stained, damaged or no longer fit.
- Donate or sell any clothing items in good condition but no longer needed.
- Store out-of-season clothing in a closet or storage container.
- Use organizers and storage solutions to keep items such as shoes and accessories tidy and accessible.

The Bathroom

- Start by removing everything from your cabinets and drawers.
- Discard any expired or unused products.

- Store towels and washcloths in a linen closet or storage container.
- Use organizers and storage solutions to keep items such as toiletries and makeup tidy and accessible.
- Invest in high-quality storage containers for cotton balls, Q-tips, and hair accessories.

The Home Office

- Start by removing everything from your desk and the surrounding area.
- Discard any outdated or unnecessary paperwork.
- Store important documents in a file cabinet or storage container.
- Use organizers and storage solutions to keep items such as pens, pencils, and paper clips tidy and accessible.
- Invest in a few high-quality storage containers for office supplies and electronic devices.

Creating a Calming Color Palette

Color plays a significant role in creating a peaceful home. Different colors can have different effects on our mood and emotions. Here are some colors to consider when creating a calming color palette in your home:

- Blue: Blue is a calming and soothing color that can promote relaxation and tranquility.
- Green: Green is a refreshing and calming color that can promote a sense of balance and harmony.
- Gray: Gray is a neutral and calming color that can create a sense of calm and serenity.

- Beige: Beige is a warm and calming color that can create a sense of comfort and relaxation.
- White: White is a pure and calming color that can create a sense of peace and tranquility.

When creating a calming color palette in your home, it's important to choose colors that make you feel relaxed and at ease. Experiment with different color combinations until you find the perfect balance for your living space.

Creating a Color Palette according to the Home Compass System

The Home Compass system has a map for optimal color placement in the home compass system. This map shows where colors feel the best and will resonate the highest in your home. Here's how it works:

- Divide your home equally into nine equal spaces in a three-by-three pattern.
- When standing at your front door, the first three colors are:
  - left - white to create a sense of connection.
  - center - blue to create a sense of creativity.
  - right - black to produce a feeling of clarity.
  - The middle section colors are:
  - left - green to promote growth and learning.
  - center - yellow to promote health and healing.
  - right - gray to encourage sharing your talents.
- The back section colors are:
  - left - purple to create a sense of luxury.
  - center - red to produce passion and warmth.
  - right - pink to create love and harmony.

Incorporating Natural Elements into Your Decor

Incorporating natural elements into your decor is a great way to create a calming and peaceful atmosphere in your home. Here are some natural elements to consider:

- Plants: Plants not only add a touch of nature to your living space, but they can also help purify the air and promote relaxation.
- Wood: Wood is a warm and natural material that can add a sense of comfort and coziness to your home.
- Stone: Stone is a natural material that can add a sense of calm and serenity to your living space.
- Water: Incorporating a water feature such as a fountain or aquarium can create a soothing and calming atmosphere in your home.

When incorporating natural elements into your decor, it's important to choose items that complement your existing decor and personal style. Feel free to experiment with different textures and materials until you find the perfect balance for your living space!

Incorporating Natural Elements into Your Decor according to the Home Compass System:

In the home compass system, we take the placements of all the natural elements a step further! Placing your elements according to the system aligns your home with the Five Element Growth Cycle of Water-Wood-Fire-Earth-Metal.

This pattern for the placement of the elements is the same as the color placement map. There's even more info in the Home Compass Workbook, but briefly, here's how it works:

- Divide your home equally into nine equal spaces in a three-by-three pattern.
- When standing at your front door, the first three elements are:
    o left - air elements like clouds, rainbows, and fans.
    o center - water elements like seashells, boats, and beach.
    o right - earth elements like stars, maps, and compasses.
- The middle section elements are:
    o left - wood elements like wood pieces, books, and games.
    o center - earth elements like salt lamps, ceramics, and pottery.
    o right - metal elements like metal pieces and artwork.
- The back section colors are:
    o left - water elements like fountains and bamboo.
    o center - fire elements like candles, lanterns, and leather.
    o right - fire elements like candles and natural light.

Maximizing Natural Light and Minimizing Artificial Light

Natural light can have a profound impact on our mood and well-being. Maximizing natural light in your home can create a sense of openness and positivity. Here are some tips for maximizing natural light in your living space:

- Keep windows clean and unobstructed.
- Use sheer or light-colored curtains to allow natural light to filter through.
- Place mirrors strategically to reflect natural light throughout your living space.
- Use light-colored paint on walls and ceilings to reflect natural light.

In contrast, artificial light can have a negative impact on our mood and sleep patterns. Minimizing artificial light in your home can create a more peaceful and calming atmosphere. Here are some tips for reducing artificial light in your living space:

- Use dimmer switches to adjust the level of light in your living space.
- Invest in high-quality light bulbs that mimic natural light.
- Avoid using harsh overhead lighting and instead opt for soft, ambient lighting.
- Use candles and other natural light sources to create a warm and inviting atmosphere.

The Benefits of Aromatherapy in Your Home

Aromatherapy is the use of essential oils to promote relaxation and well-being. Incorporating aromatherapy into your home can profoundly impact your mood and emotions. Here are some of the benefits of aromatherapy:

- Reduced stress and anxiety.
- Improved sleep quality.
- Increased energy and focus.
- Enhanced mood and emotional well-being.

Here are some ways to incorporate aromatherapy into your home:

- Use a diffuser to disperse essential oils throughout your living space.
- Add a few drops of essential oils to your bath or shower.
- Use essential oils to create a relaxing and calming massage oil.
- Use essential oils to create a calming and soothing atmosphere in your bedroom.

Any essential oils you love can help create a peaceful atmosphere in your home. Home Compass also has some essential oil blends in the Home Compass Workbook for different purposes. You can find these and more in the Home Compass Workbook available on Amazon.

Maintaining a Peaceful Home

Creating a peaceful home is an ongoing process. Here are some tips for maintaining a peaceful living space:

- Stay organized: Clutter can quickly accumulate, so it's important to stay on top of it.
- Clean regularly: Regular cleaning can help keep your home feeling fresh and inviting.
- Incorporate relaxation practices: Incorporate relaxation practices such as meditation or yoga into your daily routine to promote a sense of calm and well-being.
- Surround yourself with positivity: Surround yourself with positive people, images, and messages to create a sense of positivity and encouragement in your home.
- Stay true to your personal style: Your home should reflect your unique style and taste. Don't be afraid to incorporate items that bring you joy and happiness.

Conclusion

Your home is your sanctuary, a place where you can relax and recharge after a long day. Creating a peaceful home is about more than just aesthetics, it's about creating a space that feels comfortable and inviting. From decluttering tips to feng shui principles, there are many ways to transform your living space into a peaceful haven. By incorporating natural elements, maximizing natural light, and minimizing artificial light, you can create a calming atmosphere in your home. So, get started today and say goodbye to stress and hello to zen vibes in your home

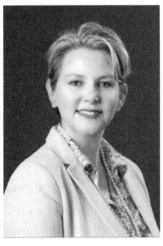

About the Author:
Kathy Watts

Kathy Watts and Home Compass's vision is for everyone to have a home space that's their happy place!

Kathy Watts is a popular speaker and teacher.

She is an idea generator, possibility detector, abundance magnet, and spontaneous creator who loves to show everyone how to have fun while doing meaningful work.

She is married with three adult children and two grandchildren.

SCAN QR CODE: Schedule to set up a Free 30-minute one on one to ask all the questions and do a mini healing protocol. Homecompass.as.me

myhomecompass.9@gmail.com

www.healyourhome.com

"Taking the 'NO'

Out of Hypnosis." ®

Chapter 13:

"Taking The Scary Out of Hypnotherapy" ®

By Shelly Jo Spinden Wahlstrom

The word "Hypnosis" elicits different emotions. Some connect it to the fun stage show they experienced either as a participant or an observer. Others think of it as "woo, woo, voodoo." And others see it for what it is: Hyper focus. It's when you are so focused on one thing that you're not paying attention to anything else.

For example: When you are driving your car and you get somewhere and wonder how you got there; or you're so focused on your phone, internet, television show and someone could be calling your name. They think you're being rude and ignoring them, and you don't even hear them. Both of those are examples of being in a hypnotic state. We go in and out of hypnosis many times throughout the day. You could almost say it's also that "daydream state."

What does it feel like? You know that feeling when you're almost asleep, but you're not. Your body feels heavy. You are aware of your surroundings, but you just don't care what's going on. Your eyes feel like they are glued shut. Your arms and legs feel so heavy that it would take too much effort to move them. It's that state of "bliss." That is what it feels like.

Yes, I'm sure you may have seen hypnosis on television where they take a pendulum and swing it in front of someone's eyes and they go into a trance. What happens is the participant or client is so focused on the pendulum that they aren't paying attention to anyone or anything around them. This causes them to go into a hypnotic state.

In your mind, there are the conscious and subconscious. The conscious part of your mind" is a small part of your thoughts, maybe 10-15% or less. This is the "I've got to get up, get dressed, go to work." It's your willpower and your goals. It's the tip of the iceberg - the part that you see. The subconscious is the part of your mind that stores every memory, emotion, and belief, you've experienced or created since you were created or before. It's the part of the iceberg - most of the iceberg- that you don't see but is below the surface of the water.

The subconscious mind's job is to keep you safe and protected. Just like a small child believes every story they are told because they have nothing to filter out whether the belief is true or false, the subconscious mind also accepts every thought or belief that it has accepted as truth. The problem is that not every story, belief or thought that is accepted is true. Because the subconscious mind's job is to keep you safe and protected, when it's trying to keep you safe and protected from a false story, that is where the problem is.

You may be able to get a small understanding of what these false beliefs and thoughts are when you listen to the words you say to yourself such as "I'm not good enough, smart enough, worthy, strong, deserving etc.". These false stories also surface when you set a financial, physical, health, or relationship goal and you find yourself sabotaging the goal. It could also be irrational fears such as fear of flying, heights, water, or even success.

What? Success? You may say, "I'm afraid of failure, but I want to succeed." Let me ask you this question. Have you ever failed before? I'm sure the answer is "Absolutely." As a child, you failed to walk on your first attempts, but you didn't stop trying to walk. In all the years I've been a hypnotherapist, I've never had one client who says that they've never failed at something. It's part of life. So, when I say you're not afraid to fail, you're actually afraid to succeed. That's different. It's easy to say you're afraid to fail but really, it's the limiting beliefs we have of what it would be like if we actually reached our goals, what would life be like? These thoughts stop us from succeeding.

Other examples of limiting beliefs would be someone who fails each time they take a test even though they know the information. Also, take for example, the athlete, performer, salesperson, or speaker who allows a negative thought into their mind after which they struggle with the activity where they normally excel.

I've had nurses and therapists who kept failing their board certifications. With hypnosis, they passed their test.

I had an athletic high school baseball player who had been playing baseball since he was a child who became afraid of the ball. Each time he'd get up to bat, he would react at the last second and miss the ball. When a ball is coming at you at 80-90 mph, that is not a good time to become afraid of the ball. The results of a hypnosis session where he made two home runs and caught the winning ball in the next game he played.

I had a talented high school cheerleader who was also a tumbler. She was proficient at doing a back tuck, until she wasn't. She had become fearful of it when she over-corrected. It was only a few weeks before the next tryouts and she had created a block that was stopping her from successfully completing a back tuck which she had been trained to do. A few days after a hypnosis session with me, her mom sent me a video showing her doing a perfect back tuck.

I've always been a seeker of truth and light. I believed in the Law of Attraction before there was "The Secret." I've always believed there's something bigger than me. I knew I wanted to be a speaker and present in a way that motivated and inspired others. I just didn't know what that would look like.

When I first heard about hypnotherapy, I had no idea how it worked. I had gone to a hypnosis show to be an observer and ended up being in the show. I remember being aware of the audience and it felt so good to be in that "blissful state" that I didn't care what was going on around me. When it was over, I felt like I was walking out in this wonderful, light cloud. I loved how it felt.

Years later, there was a man, Dennis Parker, who lived in my neighborhood who had a hypnotherapy school. I was intrigued at first, but it wasn't the right timing, until it was. When I attended my first class and watched him hypnotize a stranger off the street whose hand shook constantly and couldn't get it to stop. I watched it go from shaking profusely to calm. I actually cried because I felt the power of hypnosis and how it could be used for good. I also learned the power of our thoughts, and something called "secondary gain." This guy was a whiteboard salesman and his hand shaking had become his sympathy calling card. Consciously or subconsciously, it helped him receive more sales. Even though we had watched it go completely away in hypnosis, he chose to keep it to receive more sales. The only way to get rid of secondary gain is to get the subconscious to buy into the fact that the behavior is no longer necessary and creates a positive belief for the subconscious to hold on to make the change that the negative behavior isn't necessary for success. However, with this, I knew this was what I wanted to learn to do so that I could help others.

One more quick story about the power of hypnosis that touched my heart and changed me forever. I had a lady come to me who had come the week before. When she came this day, the first thing she said to me was "This isn't a good day. I should have canceled. I don't know if this is going to work today." When I asked her why, she said that it was her daughter's seventeenth birthday and she had passed away only after living for three days. She said that every year for the four days from the day she was born to the day she died, she did anything she could to forget and not feel the pain.

Out of my mouth came these words. "This is going to be the best day of your life." I gasped and prayed that this would be true. I had no idea where this was going to go and how I could make that promise. As we got started, one technique is to get them back in their memory before the event so you can move forward and through the trauma. She wouldn't. Each time we got close to the thoughts of her death, she kept saying "I don't know." She wouldn't go around it. All the energy was stopped on that day. It was like there were no memories before that date. Its "parts" your life and energy get blocked.

Finally, out of the blue, I said "Tell me about you baby." She said, "what did you say?" I said "Tell me about your baby. She lived for three days. Tell me about your baby." She sat there for a moment, then she lit up and proceeded to tell me about her baby; how beautiful she was, perfect, alert. Suddenly she stopped and said "Wow, I've been so focused on her death I forgot to be grateful for her life." She instantly changed. She decided from that point forward, she would celebrate her daughter's life and the special time she spent with her on this earth.

The really awesome thing was, this year on her daughter's birthday, I received a text from her saying,

"Today is my daughter's birthday and I'm celebrating." That's the power of what hypnosis can do when you get to the root of what is keeping you blocked.

In my book "FEED YOUR BRAIN - CHANGE YOUR LIFE, Take Control of Your Brain, Body, and Emotions available on Amazon, I talk about how to do self-hypnosis. Here's a synapsis of it:

1. Think about the change you want. Write down the lie and the truth of it.
2. Find a place you can go to be completely quiet and undisturbed.
3. Set a time limit. State in a suggestion, "In ten minutes I'll awake feeling refreshed."
4. Close your eyes, breathe deeply, and focus on relaxing each body part.
5. Countdown from ten to one, visualize stepping down ten steps.
6. Allow yourself to go deeper into a trance. You may feel like you're floating.
7. Once in that relaxed state, bring up the negative story or blocks you want to change.
8. Once that story has come forward, release the old story, and replace it with new thoughts.
9. Trust your subconscious to change your thoughts (software) and visualize the change.
10. Visualize going back up the steps. Reinforce the change. Feel gratitude, peace, and joy.

"Shelly is a master hypnotherapist with vast knowledge and experience. She has assisted me many times to improve and upgrade my belief system that has allowed me to become the person I am today! I continue to draw from her professional and empathic work to improve myself and live my higher self. I have recommended her to many friends and associates that also want to live a better life, and I lovingly recommend her to you! Be your best self and soar!" ~Athena~

"Anyone who's lived very long has probably faced some challenges that have wrenched their souls. Though the pathway beyond such experiences requires a great deal of personal work, it's often the case that the help of a highly skilled professional is also needed. Shelly is such a person. I was skeptical of hypnotherapy but having been stuck in my own growth for some time, I decided to give it a try. With understanding and compassion, Shelly skillfully guided me through one of the most profound and cathartic experiences of my life and I was finally able to move past my pain, press forward and find joy again. I can't thank her enough." ~John~

One of my favorite quotes is "Every day and in every way, I'm getting better and better." (Emile Coue'). Learn how to take control of your words and thoughts and you will change your life. If you want help, reach out to me. Hypnosis can be done online as effectively as in person. Once your eyes are closed, it doesn't matter where you are.

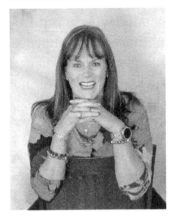

About the Author
Shelly Jo Spinden Wahlstrom, CHT, CRNC

Shelly Jo a.k.a "The Amino Acid Lady and Hypnotherapist" is a Certified Hypnotherapist; Certified Addiction, Recovery, and Mental Health Nutrition Coach.

She is currently working on her Doctorate in Metaphysics from the University of Sedona in AZ.

Shelly Jo is the Owner of Shelly Jo Hypno Aminos Nutrition - a.k.a. brain food (voted - Top 25 Coolest Things Made in Utah - Best Natural Products - Standard Examiners - Best of Northern Utah - Best Hypnotherapy Service).

She is a Best-Selling Author - "Feed Your Brain, Change Your Life - Take Control of Your Brain, Body, and Emotions."

She is an International Speaker and Presenter. She teaches a Basic Amino Acid & Nut0rition Course for practitioners interested in adding amino acids and nutrition to their practice.

Shelly Jo is the Chairperson of the Alliance for Addiction Solutions.

She lives in Utah with her husband, three amazing daughters and sons-in-law and favorite eleven grandchildren.

She is an avid skier, dancer, and player with grandchildren. Her favorite name is "Grama Shelly."

 **SCAN QR CODE: Quiz, Website, to Connect:**
Hypnoaminos.com
801-643-3211
shellyjo@hypnoaminos.com

linktr.ee/shellyjohypno

Could Amino Acids Be YOUR Missing Link

"In the Storm's Embrace,

Discovering Serenity and Unwavering Presence."

Chapter 14:

Living in the Eye of the Storm

By Tam Pendleton

FIRST OF ALL...

Can we define the term energy medicine? As simply as possible, energy medicine is the law that governs the healthy vibration of the atoms, comprising our body's cellular structures. Traumatic experiences can damage the natural health of our tissues, impairing the vibration or frequency of those atoms within the body. (We're talking about quantum theory here). Interruptions in the body's energy system, (a.k.a., the chakras and meridian vessels), may lead to medical, mental, and spiritual disorders. Using the energy tools of Love and Light, we can bring the body back into balance and alignment. It is as simple as thinking a happy thought, and therefore, too easy for the greater population to consider a viable option. Still,

141

by small and simple things are great things brought to pass.

Slammed in the storm...

Pain can be an intense catalyst for change, and finding relief from pain has been a driving force in most of my life's defining moments.

As a little girl, I struggled with a longing for home...a home beyond this earth...a home offering more safety and peace than I was able to feel with my parents. Some part of me knew I had lost my *real* home, that place from *before,* where I knew that I was precious to God. I was feeling completely out of sorts on this crazy planet. I had very young parents who were just out of high school and were experiencing a very tumultuous, drama driven, conflict-habituated relationship. By the age of twenty-three, my mother had three babies and a miscarriage in their first four years together. My dad was buried in the frustration of debt with medical bills from three caesarian births, a wife whose needs were a complete mystery to him, plus the usual life pressures with a family. These were good people trying hard to make it all work, but it didn't take long for their marriage to crumble.

As a baby, I can remember knowing that my mom could not meet my day-to-day needs, I believed that I would need to take care of her. That was overwhelming to me and laid the groundwork for some profound codependent beliefs. In my heart, I was longing for that familiar place where I was safe with my Heavenly Father. Lying in bed at night, I would fervently recite the words from a plaque next to my bed:

Now I lay me down to sleep,

I pray the Lord my soul to keep.

If I should die before I wake,

I pray the Lord my soul to take.

I would open my eyes in the morning feeling disappointed that God had not taken me back.

By the time I was eight, my parents were legally separated. The ache within deepened as I mourned the loss of my family, feeling torn between my parents' demands, along with the grief and the condemnation coming from the in-laws over the scandal of divorce. Keep in mind, our big wonderful extended family was the secret source that made everything great for me. My parents' divorce disaster threatened my *happy places*, the security I felt with the family members who kept me safe. Ironically, among those I treasured most, I was trapped in adult secrets; having been violated by a sexual predator who was hiding in my extended family.

I effectively blocked the molestations from my mind, never telling anyone. For years beyond childhood, I had violent, vivid nightmares about a perpetrator, never able to see his face. My mind had hidden the ghastly details until I was safe in young adulthood, with children of my own. Only then did those experiences come flooding back to the mind, challenging my sanity, while explaining why I had been paralyzed by sadness, dysfunction, and years of clinical depression. A powerful voice of warning and encouragement spoke to me during those years, inviting me to learn from the depths of my pain. I knew that in the future, after my own healing, thousands of people would find peace from my experience as they pursued their own. By the time I was thirty-one, married with four littles of my own, there was a reprieve from the worst of it; I had passed the gauntlet of agony and hopeless depression.

Learning to live in the eye of the storm...

The road to healing was the experience of a lifetime. Definitely, it was the hardest thing I had ever done. An unexpected spiritual strength and an understanding of the healing power of Jesus Christ widened the breadth of my soul. This knowledge expanded exponentially as a new opportunity arose. My husband and I were told through prayer that we needed to leave our California home and move, lock, stock, and barrel to Utah. We were not told why we were moving; the message was simple; move, buy a home, find a job, and go. In a matter of weeks, we carried the boxes of our belongings through the front door of our new home in Salt Lake City. It was a happy time!

The following day, we learned that a dear friend of ours (we'll call Ann), was released from a mental health hospital following a suicide attempt. She moved in with us right away. The mystery of the move was solved. We realized that God moved our whole family so that we would be in a position to love and care for Ann. Our friends and family were critical of our decision, but we knew that we were following the heavenly direction and doing the right thing. It was very humbling to think about it; Father in Heaven loved our friend so much that He moved an entire family so that she could have exactly what she needed at that critical time in her life. I realized that if He loved Ann that much, then He loves all of us that much, and miracles are provided for His people.

For four years, Ann struggled through the pain of her recovery from sexual trauma, in and out of hospitalizations, the integration of Dissociative Identity Disorder (DID), and Bipolar Disorder. At times it was a living nightmare. She was furious with God and hell-bent on destroying herself. Ann's mind had many self-abusive, wounded personalities that required therapy and protection.

As Ann's caregiver, I was at every doctor's appointment and psychotherapy session. I regulated all of her medication and watched over her every day. I loved her as one of my children, and she became part of the family. Although I was a hot mess myself and not equipped with the proper education to facilitate her healing journey; tools, and skills were given to me at the time to keep her safe. I was tutored in the healing arts, specifically to support Ann's needs. At the end of those four years, God spoke to us again, and we moved back to our California home. Ann and I continued our work together remotely for another eight years.

In the end, what I really learned was this...

` Jesus passed through the depths of our pain. He knew Ann, and He loved her. He could heal all of the trauma and the twenty-plus personalities that had splintered within her, if she would let him. Though it took many years, Ann recovered and returned to her family. She is a living reminder to me that we are God's beloved children, and he will stop at nothing to retrieve us from our own private hell.

There are many miracles in that story. First, that somehow, I married a compassionate man who refused to give up on me, and our friend Ann. Thank you, Don. And secondly, the path of my experiences led me to a deep understanding of the loving compassion of a living God and his angels who supportively minister to us daily.

In my late forties, after my youngest child had started school, I went back to school myself, and became a licensed massage therapist, life coach, and energy medicine practitioner. I loved the work of assisting a clientele who had suffered severe abuses of all kinds including emotional, physical, and spiritual wounds. Though the client's results were very good, I was searching for something that would release more complex energy structures, as well as to empower the client with mentoring tools that would carry them beyond their old habits and patterns of dysfunction.

I had been asking God for information on how to combine what I knew about healing with whatever it was I did not yet *remember*... basically what I had forgotten from *before* I came here. I wanted to remember my pre-earth gifts and to know the next step that heaven had planned for me. There was a strong feeling that whatever would come to me would profoundly impact the lives of my clients.

146

Sure enough...the moment came at 4:00 am on a June morning in 2013. As I heard my name called, waking me, I grabbed a pen and captured the download as it burst into my mind. I wrote for hours, then days. All in all, it took about two weeks to receive the outline of this new tool. I was told that this gift was the answer I had prayed for, and that this information was meant to be shared with others. There it was, the Healer's Blueprint (™) was born, and I was the steward.

Now, more than ten years later, this amazing modality has been taught to hundreds of practitioners, impacting thousands of struggling individuals; soothing minds, spiritual wounds, and bodies wracked with pain while empowering them through the Light of Christ.

Whether we like it or not...

Our lives are filled with choices about how we will perceive the experiences that come to us. We decide how to feel about what has happened. It could be a hot-mess story of tragedy or a brilliant exercise on the road to learning faith, compassion, and love; we decide.

Drama, trauma, and crazy surround all of us! Our minds will establish deep connections with the body and spirit, while trying to make sense of the life story unfolding all around us. Our life stories are literally recorded in the cells and tissues of our body. Emotional wounds are hidden, stinging within our organs and tissues. Eventually our subconscious mind will begin to manifest the broken beliefs and literally transform them into physical maladies in the body. In other words, our minds take the sad stories of our lives and convert them into physical reality.

In these tumultuous times, it can feel as if we live in the eye of a Category 5 hurricane. The perimeter of the storm is fast-moving, but inside, the winds are calm, and the pelting rain has stopped. If we keep moving at the storm's speed, we stay in the eye, even at a profound limp, and we can keep pace with the storm. But if we lag behind and are overtaken by the storm's raging bands of energy, then our own energy is spent being tossed about like an umbrella in the wind, with no strength left for caring for our own needs and the needs of those we love.

Like the analogy of the storm, our spirit-mind-body connection weakens under the stress and pressures of life, wearing us down until we fall into patterns of dis-ease and dis-integration of well-being. The answer? We wake ourselves! We level up and receive a new awareness. We start paying attention to what is happening within, and we *practice mindfulness.*

Wake-Up Action Steps:

Here are a few practical tips for mindfully living in alignment and full connection:

- BODY – Give yourself a chance to feel well and perform well everyday by doing some basic self-care for yourself, such as: quality vitamin & mineral supplementation, great sleep, movement, and eating whole unprocessed foods. Make small healthy moves, one day at a time. Without basic, nutrient rich nourishment and care, your body will be unable to survive the storms and stresses of our day.

- MIND – Find meaningful meditation moments, either guided visualizations or pondering after prayer. Give your mind a powerful peaceful location to visit, or better yet, invite God in that power space with you. Let Him heal your wounds, nurture you and help you mend as you spend meaningful time with the Creator. (Download a free visualization at TamPendleton.com)

- SPIRIT – When your heart is hurting, or anxiety, grief, panic or overwhelm threatens to overtake you, try putting one hand over your heart (heart chakra) and one hand over your lower belly (sacral chakra). Focus on the emotion moving through you, notice it, listen to it. Observe the feelings that move through you, with compassion. Speak out loud, specifically acknowledging the emotion. For example, *even though I feel angry and sad, I choose to love and to accept myself just as I am.* Then allow your heart to open wider and receive the spirit message of love. With practice, as you learn to listen, that message will surely come.

Testimonials:

"After two years of learning bits and pieces about energy work, I decided to jump in and see what it really is and if it had a place in my life. The Healer's Blueprint was the right beginning class for me – easy to understand, easy (with practice) to apply, and thorough in content. The high quality of the presentation and materials reflect the excellence of the program. And Tam Pendleton, the teacher and founder, is truly inspiring as she teaches the God-given principles that underlie this beautiful guide to healing. In my senior year, I realized it's not too late to make a difference in this wonderful world, a useful contribution to the lives of my loved ones and others, and that is exciting and invigorating to me! I can hardly wait to put into practice this simple, beautifully organized, and comprehensive plan for healing. From the bottom of my heart, I am so grateful to have been guided to the Healer's Blueprint. It has given me a new purpose in life." -Norma T.

"The Healer's Blueprint is an encompassing tool, allowing for all modalities while combining them for the most thorough and efficient use of time and subconscious allowance. My sessions with my partners have cleared immense hurdles within me, unfettering my power to be wholly unleashed. Tam is a brilliant mentor, healer, and traveler." -Nicole S.

"Being part of the Healers Academy was one of the most transformative experiences I've ever had. I found myself surrounded by like-minded people (even though I'm a 29-year-old male and I expected to feel like the odd man out). The academy and the Healers Blueprint modality have helped me to open up to my gifts and strengths in a way that I didn't think was possible. Tam is an inspired leader and teacher. I've never had an interaction or online class with her that wasn't well thought out, guided by a higher power, and deeply. meaningful to me." -Kyson K.

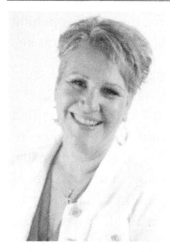

About the Author:
Tam Pendleton

Tam Pendleton was born and raised in Redlands, CA, and graduated from Redlands High. (Go Terriers!) She has practiced bodywork and energy medicine since 2007. Working with thousands of clients, she loves to facilitate others with building mind-body-spirit alignment and recovery from trauma and abuse. Her practice is focused on empowering spiritual healing and restoring a divine connection for those with religious-based wounds and difficulties in their relationship with God.

Tam has pioneered healing methods using energy healing combined with deep hypnosis to enable clients to move on from codependent relationship difficulties and traumatic experiences.

The founder of the Healer's Blueprint, Tam shares a powerful energy modality, marrying intuitive energy medicine/psychology with practical life skills. Her formula for healing uses principles of quantum mechanics, energy, and Christian values, teaching others to identify and release painful patterns of anxiety, trauma, and abuse from the body's cellular structures.

A skilled trainer, her Healer's Academy, offers an empowering international mentoring program for energy students and practitioners from across the world--opening the doors of self-love and empowerment for her clientele.

Tam has an Associate's Degree (AA) degree from Ricks College. She is a Licensed Massage Therapist (LMT), Cellular Release Therapist (CRT), Board Certified Traditional Naturopath (BCTN), and the co-owner of Integrating Wellness Center in Springville. Additionally, she has studied Craniosacral therapy, and Traditional Chinese Medicine and loves homeopathy. Tam loves to garden, cook, and travel. She is a wife of 43 years, the proud mama to five great-kids, and the "Mimi" to her beautiful grandbabies.

SCAN QR CODE:
TamPendleton.com
Email: Talkingtotam@gmail.com

"Thriving is Not Merely Surviving, But Flourishing With Radiant Vitality."

Chapter 15:

Wired to Thrive:
How to Rewire your Brain from
Surviving to Thriving

By LaMonte Wilcox

T here was a time when my life looked great from most perspectives, until my eyes were opened, and I found it was actually characterized by mental chaos. I felt constant pressure and stress because of my own mental health challenges that I was mostly unaware of. Some of my family members also struggled and I was at a complete loss. Each of us wrestled with something, and despite the love we felt for each other, we were struggling to connect and support each other's challenges in effective ways. In fact, our attempts at solving our problems only seemed to worsen them. I turned to positivity as a survival instinct *and even though I was really good at it, there were no sustainable or lasting results. I was only dodging the pain, which, over time, only seemed to increase it.*

Since the mental health system was failing my family, I began searching elsewhere for answers. I spent every spare moment researching the latest discoveries in neuroscience and psychology. I resonated deeply with what I was learning. After discovering the concept of neuroplasticity, I realized that we could, as a family, rewire our responses to each other and to our own inner emotional states. I began developing and practicing techniques based on what I was learning. I was blown away by the powerful and lasting shifts I was seeing in myself and my family. It wasn't long before our entire family life and relationships were completely transformed!

I knew other families would benefit from learning this. I wanted to make this my life's work. I began using these techniques to reprogram my own thinking around work and soon left my twenty-year career in sales so I could devote myself full-time to this new rewarding experience.

I shared what I was learning with a functional medicine neurologist who ran a Neuro-wellness Clinic. After seeing amazing results with a few of his patients, the doctor, to my great delight, invited me to open an office in his clinic so I could work with some of his most challenging patients, those who struggled with treatment-resistant mental illnesses and addictions.

As I began seeing consistent transformations in these clients, I became excited about refining the model I had developed to help people reprogram their brains – breaking longstanding 'dysfunctional' patterns of relating, thinking, and feeling that had kept them stuck in unsatisfying situations and in the grips of unrelenting mental distress for many years.

I spent two years at the clinic working with a wide range of people who had a variety of mental and physical health challenges, even those with TBI's (Traumatic Brain Injuries). After a year, my daughter McKelle joined me. This model was helping even those with conditions that were thought to be lifelong pervasive illnesses like: schizophrenia, bipolar, and personality disorders. Even addictive behaviors were diluted in only one session!

As I watched transformation after transformation, I became more excited and wanted to reach even more people. So, I left the clinic, and along with my daughter, who had quickly embraced these concepts and shared my desire to help as many as possible, developed the F.L.Y. (Fulfill Life Yourself) Neuro-wellness Program.

It's a self-paced online program that teaches the model and provides specific activities and exercises that rewire the brain. The program works because it teaches you to go deep into the concepts of how the brain works and gives you daily activities and assignments that break down old mind maps. This naturally results in the elimination of stubborn patterns, behaviors, and mental challenges. As your conscious mind begins to interact differently with your subconscious mind, you are literally rewiring your brain, allowing for major shifts and changes in your life.

I've noticed that most of the attempts to help people with mental illnesses focus on relieving symptoms and improving daily functioning, instead of getting to the core and resolving the blocks that prevent them from creating a life of joy, peace, and happiness. Learning how to access these inner states powerfully affects a person's neurotransmitters and provides much more than symptom relief. It transforms a person's whole way of seeing, thinking, and feeling.

As individuals develop an awareness and understanding of how their brain is either working for them or against them at any given moment, it gives them the true power of choice allowing them to shift from old programming into the freedom of creating something new - the life they truly want.

I've witnessed this transformation hundreds of times in the lives of my clients, and this is only one of many client's stories, written in her own words:

"I started having seizures when I was 6 years old. Despite many visits to many different doctors and many tests and procedures, doctors could not find a cause. They just prescribed medications that sometimes didn't work or had terrible side effects. My parents tried everything – herbal and homeopathic remedies, the Keto diet, medical marijuana, and all kinds of therapies. Nothing worked.

As a young adult, I felt thwarted and became more and more depressed. I developed an obsessive-compulsive disorder, thinking that in some strange way I might be able to control the things that caused me to have seizures, but instead of controlling them, I started feeling them coming on constantly.

I had married a man who was very understanding of my limitations, yet our relationship was becoming more strained as I continued to become more debilitated. I started having anxiety and panic attacks every time I got up from the couch or bed. It got to the point where I couldn't get up from the bed or couch without an attack. Because of this, I demanded a lot from the people around me, including my husband. I couldn't seem to find a way out despite trying so many different things. I began seriously considering suicide, sometimes on a daily basis, because I just couldn't keep living like this.

One day, my mom came over and shared the F.L.Y. neuro-wellness program with me. On the very first day of doing the program, I was able to get up and go outside for a little while. I was definitely "sold," and continued doing it. The changes were remarkable. I began doing more and more for myself - cooking, folding laundry, even driving!

Seven months after I started the program, I was totally free of depression, anxiety, and seizures. I never had another thought of suicide. I'm on a very low dose of medication and the OCD is mostly gone! I will be forever grateful for this program because it taught me that we have the power to take charge of our brains and our bodies, if shown how.

Not only was my physical and mental health restored, but my marriage was saved and relationships with my family improved dramatically!" – Julia Kellerstrass.

If you are a person, like Julia, who has been trying for many years to overcome some type of challenge – whether it's an addiction, mental health symptoms, relationship issues, parenting challenges, or some other area where you feel blocked or stuck – I highly recommend learning about how your brain works.

You'll discover how conditioned, or wired, we are to respond to stimuli in our environment in certain predictable ways. This subconscious programming starts early with our family, our religion, the media, politics, culture, and the institutions that seek to influence or control us. This internal programming continues to impact how we think about and perceive ourselves, others, and how the world works. It will continue exerting its influence over us until we learn how to break free from it. Only then can we exercise true agency and have the power of choice.

Understanding how your brain works can greatly enhance the results of other healing modalities, allowing these to affect you on a deeper level. Another powerful way to help change your brain's programming is by listening to the stories of individuals who have already overcome challenges like yours. This opens up possibilities within and helps you stay focused on what you are moving toward, instead of being afraid of or opposing what you are trying to move away from.

Hope is the catalyst to change. Distraction will be your biggest obstacle. The F.L.Y. Neuro-Wellness Program is designed to keep new neuro experiences going strong and long enough to stick, until they become second nature, completely replacing old programming, and removing the need to discipline ourselves towards your goals. It will become your nature to move towards the behaviors that lead you to a life of true success and happiness.

As you learn what is really driving your thoughts and behaviors, your old beliefs will be challenged. For some patterns, it will take some fortitude to continue this self-discovery and forward momentum toward the life you want. For others, you can find immediate life-changing results. If you continue, however, you'll find a higher purpose and a deeper meaning of empowerment that you never knew was possible.

Here are three steps you can take today to begin the self-reprogramming process. To get the most from this experience, actually write the answers down.

- **First**, notice that every experience you have is just a series of connections in your brain, like in the movie The Matrix. They are all just trying to get chemical needs met. When your brain developed as a child, it learned how to process its perception of things in a way that met its chemical needs. Now answer this question: If this really is true, what could you change now in your life?

- **Second**, realize that your reality is not what it seems, so question your perceptions and beliefs that were programmed into you as your brain developed (ages birth to 7). Most, especially the ones that make you feel the feelings that you don't like to have. (Shame, disappointment, procrastination, depression, anxiety, fear, frustration, anger, jealousy, etc. Any feeling you wouldn't choose to have, you don't have to experience. Now, if this is true, what experiences would you change today?

- **Third**, search for a different perspective that helps you experience a feeling that you want. Love, peace, joy, enthusiasm, connection, clarity, excitement, celebration, are great options. Find a possible outcome that even excites you. You may have to look far into the future to realize that a current experience is going to help you achieve your goals. This often takes some examples and practice.

We are here to help if you need it. If done effectively, like the scene in The Matrix you will start to see the algorithms behind your perception and begin to take control of your experience and help your brain achieve the chemical balance it needs in ways that help you move closer to your ultimate goals. You have just achieved true fulfillment!

You can either go and research and learn all the latest discoveries in neuroscience and psychology to change your own patterns, or you can learn from my experience by contacting me directly. (Methods to contact me are on the end of my biography)."

You'll learn how to give, love, and create from a higher level. In the end, it's all about learning how to clear out old programming so you can access your true inner guidance system which is built into each of us and contains all truth – the truth that leads to pure joy, peace, love, and true fulfillment, our highest creation - our life experience!

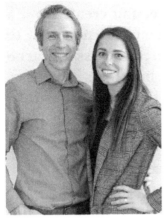

About the Author:
LaMonte Wilcox

LaMonte Wilcox, along with his daughter McKelle, teaches therapists, social workers, healers, life coaches, parents, and anyone who struggles with mental health challenges or addictions, the F.L.Y. (Fulfill Life Yourself) Neuro-wellness model he developed.

This model empowers people, in only a few visits, to take control of their neurochemical balance through a deep understanding of how their brain works, thus resolving the core cause of their suffering and opening the door to true fulfillment.

LaMonte has been invited to lecture at local universities, conferences, and to educators and other groups. He shares research on how modern lifestyles, especially technology, affect the brain and how this correlates to increasing mental illnesses.

He is one of the co-founders of a non-profit, The Living Well Project, whose mission is to help young people counteract the effects of technology that can lead to depression, anxiety, and suicidal thoughts.

He is the founder of Fulfill Life Yourself, LLC (F.L.Y.), a mental health coaching organization with a vision to empower this generation to levels of mental success and healing that can change the world.

He created the FLY Facilitator program that provides the opportunity for clients who have experienced their own transformation to be trained to share the model with others while earning an income to support the lifestyle they desire. This consistent exposure helps them continue to apply the principles and thus accelerates them to a much higher potential.

SCAN QR CODE:
FullfillLifeYourself.com
Follow his YouTube Channel at
YouTube
Email: FLY@FulfillLifeYourself.com
Phone: 801-405-3321

"Within Each Moment,

Healing Choices Shape Our Journey."

Chapter 16:

Time Does Not Heal All Wounds, You Do!

By Suzi Bell

nyone who enters the field of healing or coaching comes from a background or had experiences of struggle where it got low enough that they were done and decided that something has to change. My story began as a child. I had very imperfect parents who were amazing. I learned to work hard, to be diligent, and to stay close to God. Yet, one thing I didn't learn was to express myself, especially the healthy expression of my feelings. I buried them.

As the Fourth child, I played small, walking in my sister's footsteps, wanting to be like them. These buried emotions didn't serve me well when I was especially sensitive and emotional. Resentment, anger, and low self-esteem built up. I love those versions of me because I didn't know better. I have compassion for those younger versions of me. She did the best she could.

I got married and carried all the buried emotions and feelings, and beliefs into my marriage. A year and a half into marriage, I found myself at a spot where I felt unloved, worthless, and broken. I didn't see anyone else around struggling like I was. It got to a point where I ran out of my apartment, hid in a small grove of trees, sat on a rock, and cried. I felt utterly hopeless that my life would get better, despite the fact I lived in paradise. I was walking into the library on campus, and my sister called me." Hi? I learned about energy healing, and I bet it would really help!" In my mind, I said, "You have no idea what I'm going through..." She was persistent. She texted, called, and emailed me.

I believe she was divinely guided to keep talking about it. Finally, I got the book for myself. I read it. I devoured it. I put it into practice. It answered questions my soul had been wanting to know before I even asked it! I learned muscle testing. I learned how to release trapped emotions. And it excited me! The prompting came to get certified. "YOU HAVE TO DO THIS" ... over and over again. I followed it, and that one decision has changed my life. I learned that healing is not something you wait for. Time does not heal all wounds. Addressing the pain and turning it into a gift so that you grow from it heals all wounds. I've learned several healing modalities, including Emotion Code, Body Code, and Foot zoning. I've attended conferences and seminars for self-improvement. I now know that my worth does not depend on my relationships, my mistakes, or my circumstances. I get to be the change agent in my life.

That is what I will help you to do. I help you to see what you really want, and I guide you into discovering what is stopping you. You might want something so bad, but you keep stopping yourself from getting it. The feelings are so strong, that the resistance wins. I take you through a simple process of questioning what is going on, understanding what it is, and releasing it. This leaves space for positive and uplifting energy to take place. Then, we elevate and empower you with tools to keep you progressing. Nourishment is the last step to becoming your best authentic, royal self. It's what helps you keep moving forward to have the energy to show up powerfully.

I have one client I want to tell you about. I will call her Jane for privacy. Jane was 8 months pregnant with her 3rd child. She had a rough pregnancy, physically and emotionally. She was terrified of giving birth in the hospital due to birth trauma with her daughter. I knew I could help her change the trajectory of her birth into one where she would be empowered and find healing in it. Her mom gave her my number, and she reached out to me. Within two sessions, we identified the glitches with her belief with her body, and released the belief that her body failed. In fact, her body saved her! That mental mindset shift changed everything for her, which led to a birth that was so healing for her. She did the steps I advised and felt better in her last 3 weeks of birth than when she had her entire pregnancy. What she wanted most was a healing birth, and we cleared away what was stopping her.

I've got another client who came to me feeling stressed out and overwhelmed. One of the things that overwhelmed her was that she didn't want to go to a resort with her family in the summer. She was invited to go two weekends in a row, one by her parents, and one by her in-laws. The emotions and beliefs behind that were because of family trauma she experienced growing up and other life decisions. What was really holding her back was that she had a hard time telling what she really wanted, the truth. She would make excuses of why she couldn't attend something where her family members would come back with a solution. We released the beliefs contributing to this and opened her mind up to what else was possible! She then communicated what she wanted on the soul level, which was that she didn't want to go because it was too stressful. Both her parents and her in-laws understood! She got the best result, while speaking her authentic truth.

I have a few tips to help you step into your power by stepping into your truth and your potential.

1. You must move out the emotion. This means expressing yourself. Find that safe person or method that helps you. If you don't have a way, journal, "I feel _____ because _____...." And then destroy it. Burn it. Tear it up. Scribble over it. Whatever helps you move out the emotion.

2. Write down what you really desire. Let go of what you fear others might be thinking or how it's not possible. Put it out into the universe!

3. Journal this question: "What step do I need to take to get this result? Who do I need to tell the truth to? And what else is possible that I am not seeing?

4. **Take action.**

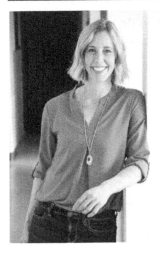

About the Author:
Suzie Bell

Suzie Bell is a mother of 4 kids, a wife, a speaker, and creator of the Arise Energy Healing System. She is a former personal trainer.

Suzie is trained in several modalities, including Emotion Code, Body Code, Energy Connections, Foot zoning, and Intuitive Mentoring.

She has many passions. She loves helping women express themselves as the best, most confident versions of themselves.

She loves birth and lights up when she helps women achieve the birth of their dreams.

The ocean is her happy place. She enjoys being in nature and trying out new things!

Her latest passion is Aerial and pole fitness! She is a master emotional release facilitator and mindset shifter.

She hosts adventure retreats and teaches the art of energy work and foot zoning so she can spread her light, love, and knowledge through her students.

SCAN QR CODE: https://aws.tini.app/
808-687-0624
Arisewithsuzie@gmail.com

"In the Realm of Dreams,

The Soul's Truth Finds Its Voice."

Chapter 17:

Whose Dream is It Anyway?

By Pamela Tolman

Not long ago, my friend asked me to speak to her group. I anxiously said "Yes." Then she asked the topic I had in my mind. I heard the words "healing the body." I was teaching this online. Out of my mouth came the words "dream therapy." WHAT?!?!?!?!?!?" When I tried to quickly retreat, she encouraged me to go with it.

A few weeks later it was time for the Zoom meeting. I was nervous, my computer was on the fritz, and I could see no one, but they could both see and hear me. To be honest, when the meeting was almost over, I didn't remember much about it. However, I remembered hearing my grandfather's voice telling me to "Be calm, to breathe, and listen to the words."

At the time, I had been taking a stage hypnosis class from a wonderful stage hypnosis friend who unbeknownst to me was in the meeting. I later received a call from him asking me why I was not doing more on dreams. I realized I had let fear overtake me and didn't believe in myself.

He spent hours with me, wanting me to see my talent and helping me to see the ability I have to help people understand their dreams.

Would you like to know more about dreams? Grab your pen and paper, find your comfortable spot, pull up your magic carpet, and take the journey into the world of dreams with me. Let me first ask you two questions:" What did you dream about last night? What are your dreams trying to tell you? These questions have been asked for centuries.

From where do dreams come? The hippocampus in the brain has the ability to remember, imagine, and is where dreams are formulated. Your dreams are molded from your thoughts, memories, and actions. Most dreams come from something that you have experienced during your waking hours. It may be thoughts that you have on your own, thoughts linked to someone else's opinion, or even a thought that may not belong to you but is stuck in your cellular memory from generations past.

The reason your dreams are not the exact thought is that they are not built from one thought or one memory, or even one experience, but from many. Your dreams are built of fragments or all your memories, experiences, and thoughts, intermingling with one another, or perhaps even the swirling effects of those thoughts going through and around each one until they fall into place as the storyline for your dream.

What Does Your Dream Mean?

There are several books that can tell you what certain things in your dreams mean. However, each one of those books is just a suggestion from someone's opinion on what they think it means. Before you go running to a bookstore to see what someone you don't even know thinks, check in with yourself first. Slow down, write it down, break it down.

If you are interested in your dreams, you may want to keep a dream journal or a notebook and pen by your bedside. When you awaken, make it a habit to write down your dreams before you ever leave your bed. The longer you wait, the more vague the dream becomes; the more intrusions and interpretations you allow into it.

Also, where were your thoughts and emotions as you drifted off to sleep? Your dreams can be fascinating, weird, frightening, or exciting. So much depends on where your emotions and thoughts were at the time you go to sleep.

Have you ever woken up from your sleep and found yourself sweating or frightened because you were being chased by someone or something in your dream? Possibly in your dream, you met someone that sparked your interest, and you want to know more about the person. Maybe you were speaking to a crowded room, and you were naked (common dream). Maybe, you were in the middle of one of "those" dreams that makes you feel so good in fact that you may have experienced what is referred to as a "wet dream".

It could be that your heart was pounding, and you could feel the blood as it rushed through your veins, the beads of sweat forming on your head and the hair on the back of your neck was standing up. Possibly, what you thought was chasing you really wasn't a person or a monster at all; instead, it was an opportunity that you couldn't make up your mind about. Could it be the reason you felt naked in front of the group was simply because you were unprepared for something? If you were to change that dream and you were to imagine all the people in the audience naked, would that thought make you feel more at ease?

Dreams can allow you to find answers to questions that you have been pondering. If there is something to which you want an answer, write that question down on the paper and place the paper beneath your pillow at night. Ask for the answers to come to you in your dreams. Again, be ready to write down your dreams in the morning, take time to review the dream, and find answers.

One of my clients was telling me about a dream she had associated with a recent date. She was positive that the dream was a sign that this was her soul mate. Yet, she felt something wasn't quite right. We took the time to break each scene of the dream down. Finally, we were only left with the music. In the background was a song that she said wasn't familiar with, but she did know it was Johnny Cash singing. The words of the song she remembered were "It ain't you babe, it ain't you. I'm looking for Babe". Still determined that her date was her soul mate, I continued to ask more questions which revealed that the waiter, in her dream, was giving her the eye and flirting with her. She thought it was rude since she was there on a date. When she described him to me, she remembered how he looked, and that he was nice.

It was no surprise to me that a couple of weeks later, she contacted me to let me know she was no longer dating the first guy but had been dating the "waiter." She was having an enjoyable time with him and thanked me for helping her to not just see what was in her dream, but to hear it as well. Sometimes when you look at your dreams, it's more than looking at them. You also need to hear what they are telling you or what may be in the background.

Another client had a reoccurring dream that she was writing a book. She had thought about writing a book several times and had even come up with the idea, and the plot, and just needed a good ending. She kept putting it off. After several nights of the same dream, it suddenly changed. She was still writing the book, only now she had a fog that would hang all around her in the dream. A few nights later in her dream, she found herself just sitting at the table, with no fog, but no book either. What happened to change the dream?

It is my belief that we receive messages in our dreams. It is up to us to search the messages for what they are telling us. I believe that she was given the message to complete her book, maybe if she would have paid better attention to the dream, the ending of the book would have come to her. Instead, when the fog was lifted, the idea for the book went with it. It is my thought that when we are given a message and fail to act upon it, that gift or message is then given to someone else who is receptive and willing to act upon it. Who knows if she would have taken the time to act, she may have a bestseller now?

Recurring Dreams:

A recurring dream is worth PAYING ATTENTION to! Is it giving you the answer to something you have been worrying about in your life?

It could be recurring because of an unresolved conflict coming from your memories, or because you have spent time being stressed about something that you aren't taking the time to recognize. What's going on in your life or around you? Breaking down dreams can be like a set of children's building blocks. You may have to build them up and take them apart to find the best solution. Connect the dots, find the structure, and figure out the meaning of the dream. You may want to begin with the obvious, review your day, and several days before the dreams start. Do they have anything in common? If so, then start building on that. What is the common factor? Is it a person, a place, a time, or a song? What is the feeling that is being brought forth? You may have to return to your past. Has there been something in your past memories that has triggered something in your present? Answer these questions in your dream notebook.

After a few nights, take some time to compare your notes and see what and where the similarities are. Once that comparison has been made, you can now start to figure out where you need to launch into the discovery and overcome any issues or move forward on the journey.

It may be that at a time in your life, you had to endure unmet needs or perhaps it was a trauma that hasn't been processed through the body. It is showing up in the dream state to get your attention before it shows up somewhere in the body as a dis-ease or injury. Dreaming is one way for your subconscious mind to speak to you. Since it will come to you in a dream, you will most likely not receive the literal words describing the event to you, but instead it will come to you metaphorically.

Let's say that you are dreaming about being on your phone and you're unable to hear the words being spoken. When you begin moving those building blocks into a pattern and the dots begin to connect, the phone may be telling you that there may be a lack of communication with someone in your life. You may want to ask yourself "Who do I need to communicate with at this time? Maybe it could be that it is a message **for** you personally, **from** you, or **about** you, that could be an aid to improving your life. It could be a message coming **to** you from a time before, if you believe in past life, or message that perhaps you failed to learn before you came to this space and you are now being given a second chance.

If you question past life, here are my thoughts and why questions may show up in your dreams. Bodies are made of protons, neutrons, and electrons which are forms of energy. When you die your energy doesn't die with you, instead is transformed. Some people look at death as the end of time, others look at it as a new beginning or a new journey. What if you were to look at it as your energy is being redistributed?

At any given moment, the body has about 20 watts of energy coursing through the body. This is enough energy to power a light bulb. You receive this energy through the consumption of food, which then gives you chemical energy. That energy is then transformed into kinetic energy, which powers your muscles. Thermodynamics has proven that energy cannot be changed or destroyed, instead, it simply changes its state. This means you have the ability to exchange your energy with your surroundings. You gain and lose energy.

When that moment of "death" takes place, the atom collection that you are made of is then repurposed. Therefore, your light is the essence of all your energy, and will continue to reverberate throughout the universe until the end of time.

Now, if all those protons, neutrons, and electrons are all traveling around, over, under, and through each species of this earth, why would you not pick up memories or thoughts of someone else's life? Since you are unaware that it is happening then it now becomes your memory, your story.

Lucid Dreams:

Lucid dreaming is nothing more than knowing that you're dreaming while you're sleeping. You understand that whatever images may be going through your brain at that time aren't really happening, regardless of how real it feels. Reaching the lucid dreaming state is just a matter of being in-between where you aren't asleep, and you're not really awake. While in a lucid dream state, you do have control over the actions that are taking place or that you are performing.

You may experience false awakening while sleeping. A false awakening is a vivid and convincing dream that you are waking up from a dream while you continue to sleep. You may feel you are performing daily tasks, taking a shower, eating a meal, or pouring yourself a cup of coffee.

You may experience the feeling of going to the bathroom. You may be dreaming about going to the bathroom and when you awaken you have wet the bed. Another type of lucid dreaming is when you are dreaming that you are having a dream. That then becomes a dream within a dream.

You may think that you ACTUALLY travel when you're lucid dreaming. You may be dreaming of traveling, but you don't really travel to any place. There are those people who wish they could lucidly dream but for one reason or another feel they can't. Let me give a few suggestions that may help.

Lucid dreaming takes place in REM sleep which is the same place all dreams happen. Being in that state of REM often will allow you to go there easily after you learn. Trusting yourself is an important factor in this journey. If you aren't getting enough sleep, it is less likely you will have the opportunity to experience any lucid dreaming. Make sure you are getting enough sleep and stop worrying about if you will or will not accomplish your goal that particular night.

By writing your dreams down in your dream journal, you are forcing your brain to recall the dream and the feelings. This will train your brain to pay attention to what you dream. This is also a time to get creative, read through your journal as often as possible to keep your brain familiarized with the dream. It also allows you to connect the dots or use the building blocks to put things into order.

You may want to set an alarm to wake you up every three to four hours after you have gone to bed. You are interrupting the dream cycle, and when you go back to sleep you will most likely enter the stage of REM sleep making it possible to enter into that long awaited lucid dream.

The easiest way would be to tell yourself several times a day that when you sleep, you have lucid dreams. You might even take the time to imagine yourself sleeping and then waking in the lucid dream state. This allows the subconscious mind to see the truth, that you easily enter into the lucid dream state.

The subconscious mind believes what it is told so let yourself become the child at play and pretend to sleep, then sometime in that pretend sleep, pretend to sleep again, or even begin to imagine yourself doing an activity in the dream, that is a dream.

There are a couple of ways to test yourself for lucid dreaming. If you were to pinch your nose closed while keeping your mouth closed, can you still breathe? If so, then you are dreaming. If you push an object through the palm of your hand, you are most likely dreaming. If you see yourself all snuggled up with a book and a blanket, and you're reading that wonderful book, take note of what you are reading, then look away. When you bring your gaze back to the book, has the story or the text of the book changed in any way?

By writing your dreams down, it can help you to see patterns in your life. It's easier to break down your dreams to find meaning if they are written down, and then you write down your discoveries as they become clear. In the dream state, you may connect with your intuition or maybe your creative side will be able to show itself more in this state of mind. If you have been struggling with your emotions, you may find that your dream is related to the processing of recent emotional memories, or emotions that you have been hiding, that are now stuck within the mind, waiting to be released.

It's important to write down your dreams as soon as you awaken. With all of modern technology, you may find that voice to text on your phone is handier than writing it all down. When you take the time to jot the dream down on paper, you may receive an image to go along with what you are describing from your dream, take a few moments to draw it out. You could decide to have a dream friend with whom you can share text messages about your dreams. This may help with dream recall. Whether it's a notebook or a friend, don't wait too long before you begin describing the dream. If you set your intention for recall before you go to bed, by telling yourself you not only want to dream but that you also want to remember what you dream your chances are once again higher.

The more consistently you record and work through your dreams, the more likely you are to understand your life better.

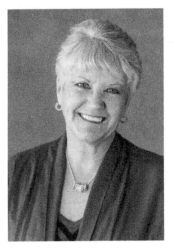

About the Author
Pamela Tolman,

Pam Tolman is a Master Certified Clinical Hypnotherapist. She began almost 30 years ago after a diagnosis of multiple sclerosis.

After this life-changing diagnosis, she focused on using hypnotherapy, meditation, and other techniques, to help her control her condition.

This change ignited a desire in her to share what she had learned to help others. Pam has spent thousands of hours educating herself, teaching others, and speaking to groups at colleges and conferences in NV, UT, WY, ID, and MT.

She owns a hypnotherapy practice and school. She is a published author of the book Hypnosis for Faster Pain Relief. Pam is an international speaker.

She considers it her personal mission to help others to release the bonds of addiction, excess weight, chronic pain, grief, anxiety, and day-to-day stress. She has had the opportunity to assist clients, friends, and family, with these issues along with feelings of TMJ, PTSD, sleep disorders, and sports.

On a couple of special occasions, Pam has helped friends with hypnobirthing. On the other side of that, she has had the opportunity to be with a family taking them through the transition as their loved one left this life for a new journey.

In her work as a clinical hypnotherapist. Pam is passionate about strengthening individuals and families by tailoring the different techniques to their needs. Thus, ensuring that each and every day is truly seen as the gift it is meant to be. Pam does more than survive; She thrives, and so can you!

SCAN QR CODE to
pamshealthandhealing.com
hypnotekniq@yahoo.com
pam@pamshealthandhealing.com
Facebook – Pam's Health and
Healing

Phone: 307-887-0138

"Essential Oils:

Nature's Aromatic Healers,

Soothing Mind and Body."

Chapter 18:

Calming Essential Oil and How to Use Them

By Kristi Corless

ave you ever felt so stressed or overwhelmed you wanted to scream? Or cry and let it all out? Did you? Good for you! We need to release those emotions. Did you know breathing has been an amazing release technique proven to calm and reduce the cortisol in the body?

When you add in the highest quality essential oils, the results get even better! When we breathe in the essential oil, it goes straight to the olfactory nerve, then to the limbic system (the emotion center of the brain), and to the rest of the body, calming or energizing and uplifting as needed in as little as 20 to 30 seconds.

With growing anxiety, stress, overwhelm, depression, and suicide rates climbing every day, more people are turning to essential oils for a natural way to calm or lift their mood without the harmful side effects. Here are some tips to remember.

Quality matters.

There is not a lot of regulation out there when it comes to essential oils which, unfortunately, this leads to adulteration. Significantly diluted oils, oils processed with pesticides and other harmful chemicals, or fragrance oils being sold as 100% "pure," these chemically altered and ineffective oils are being passed off as healthy and effective. Not only are they not giving the desired results, but they can also be harmful.

When I first became a foot zonologist, I used different brands of oils, and I had tried a few different kinds. When I was introduced to a high-quality essential oil (Look in my bio to see the essential oils I recommend), I could tell the purity and potency immediately. I could tell it was the best quality I'd tried, by smelling the peppermint! The nose knows! I found out they do over 50 tests per batch to guarantee the best quality and effectiveness with every bottle. I've been using them and teaching about the benefits ever since. As I share information in this chapter, it's my recommendation to achieve the best results, find an essential oil that is of the highest and purist quality, and has been tested, and can be trusted.

Three ways to use them.

One of the best ways to use essential oils for calming or uplifting the mood is by breathing them in, or what we call **"aromatic."** You can add it to a diffuser to disperse into a room. Place a drop in one palm and rub together with the other, cup hands over nose and inhale for 7 to 10 deep breaths. Repeat as needed for calming. You can also try a few drops on a foot soaked in some Epsom salt. If you love baths and your muscles also need calming add 1-2 cups of Epsom salt to a bath with 5 to 7 drops of oil. Side note, Magnesium found in those Epsom salts is very calming for stress, pain, and mopping up excess toxins, so soak in those Epsom salts with the added calming effect from the oils as often as you can.

Internal use may also be safe if using a medicinal grade oil. Sometimes Frankincense or Melissa taken internally over time have helped with deep feelings of sadness. I experienced this. I had gone through infertility, adoption, IVF, and had our last child on our own! My business was thriving! Yet, I felt as if nothing I did was good enough and I was in a pit. I felt overwhelmed, heavy, and stuck and couldn't rise out of it. I finally had everything I wanted, yet I felt empty inside, and no success was enough. After using a high-quality vitamin and incorporating Frankincense and Melissa, mostly aromatically and internally throughout my day, I felt as though I was lifted right out of that pit, and I was walking on water!!!!

#1 **Lavender:** when in doubt, pull your Lavender out! This is my first oil because of its well-known use in aromatherapy. And boy does it have the science to back it up too! It's probably the most commonly used and most well-known oil around the world. It's known for "all things calming" acting as a natural antihistamine to calming inflammation, stress, and anxiety, calming burns on the skin, or other skin rashes, bruises, scrapes and minor wounds. Even helpful for shock, and grief. Got head tension? Try applying a drop or two of lavender **topically** (means on top of the skin) to the area of concern.

You can look up study after study on pub med. Type in the oil and what you want to know. For example, "Lavender and stress reduction" or "Lavender and reduced anxiety." It truly is the Swiss army knife of essential oils. It's also known in the energetic & emotional properties as the oil of "communication" Specifically calming the insecurities felt when one risks their true thoughts and feelings. It will help you go from Unheard-to-Expressed.

#2 **Frankincense** comes in as my number two for calming. Even though it could also be considered #1.

It's a great one for enhancing meditation, or prayer. Use a diffuser to clear/cleanse a room of negative/low energy. Apply it on the third eye or over the heart, under the nose or the back of neck. Also great for anxious feelings, especially when trauma involving the brain is concerned, like TBI. It can calm the issues related to that. Cup and inhaling aroma from palms of hands is so powerful. It calms the brain so it can focus better too. It's such a powerful oil, no wonder it was good enough to make the cut; for the wise men to give to baby Jesus.

The emotions and energetic insights: Considered the oil of Truth. It reveals false truths, and deceptions. Invites us to let go of lower vibrations of sadness, lies, negativity, etc. Frankincense supports a healthy relationship with one's father and the Divine Father... It helps individuals feel the love of the divine. It helps shield yourself from negative influences. It's good for kids who have night terrors or nightmares. Diffuse or keep by the bed to apply if needed. You can use it on the bottom of feet, back of the neck, over the heart. It helps you move from "Separated to Unified."

#3 **Magnolia** is next on my list. It smells absolutely amazing and reminds me of a lilac tree.

Magnolia can be used "as mentioned," in a bath, breathed in, or diffused around the home. It's also a great one to apply in a clockwise motion over your lower abdomen, wrists, or ankles for help with hormonal imbalances, cramps, etc. Specifically great for anger, rage, irritability, panic, shock, grief, and sadness. Feeling stressed, uptight or tense? Worried, have a low sex drive? Or maybe insomnia? This is another one to try if Lavender doesn't do the trick.

It's the oil of compassion. Helps with a broken heart, and the ability to receive love. Connecting us with the Divine Matriarch. Nurturing, loving, and inviting, the sweetness of Magnolia draws the senses in with gentle pure maternal nurturing that facilitates deep soul-level healing and change. Emotionally go from Disturbed to Confident.

#4 **Rose** could also be a #1 oil. Rose carries the highest vibration of all essential oils on the planet. Great hormone

191

balancing like PMS, irregular ovulation, menstruation, and miscarriage. It is a powerful healer of the heart and helps connect us with Divine Love. This love reminds us it heals all hearts and dresses all wounds. Another great choice for meditation because it is such a great natural sedative. Apply topically under the nose, wrists, back of neck, or bottom of feet. Great in a massage diluted with coconut oil or another carrier oil. It opens the heart to receive. Emotionally, you can go from Isolated to feeling loved.

#5 **Melissa** is one of my favorites for uplifting the mood and feelings of anxiousness. When I struggled with depression, breathing it in aromatically several times a day and placing a drop behind the ears worked well. Also, I took a drop on or under my tongue a few times a day. If you don't love the smell, simply add a citrus or another favorite oil with it as you breathe it in aromatically.

Melissa awakens the soul to truth and light. Reminds individuals who they are and why they came to this earth. Helps you release anything and everything not in alignment with reaching your fullest potential! See why I love it?! Depressed-Light filled!!!

My favorite calming oil blend has wild orange, lavender, copaiba, spearmint, magnolia, rosemary, neroli, and sweet gum. Adaptiv® is from doTERRA® and contains all of these in one blend. It helps our body.

Coming back to topical use, there was a teenager who experienced intense anxious feelings daily. Her first Prom was only a week away and she was on her period. When I saw her, she was panicking and sobbing, almost hysterical... I didn't think I could foot zone her. I couldn't get her up to my massage table for the "Aromatouch back technique", however, I could sit next to her on the floor. So, one by one, I placed the drops of each of those oils up her spine, from the base of her spine to the base of her skull. I watched her go from completely overwhelmed to calm within about 5 to 10 min. It was "SO POWERFUL!!!

Who do you know who needs these powerful tools in their tool belt?

References:

"Essential Emotions" – Essential Emotions, LLC."

"Essential Life" – Total Wellness Publishing

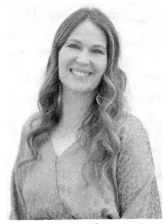

About the Author:
Kristi Corless

Kristi Corless has 4 beautiful children ages 12, 13, 17, and 20.

She has an amazing supportive husband.

She struggled with infertility(endometriosis) and adopted 2 children, 1 came through in vitro and 1 the "old fashioned." way after finding natural answers to her challenges.

She realized her purpose and mission was to help others find natural healing solutions too. She has been sharing and educating through the vehicle of dōTERRA®, with their unparalleled products for over 12 years.

She has 13 years of experience and 10 certifications in alternative healing methods including foot, back, face, and hand zoning. Access bars, Reiki, Bones I, Bones II (deep emotional releasing) the Aromatouch back technique. She's a certified Life coach. She created her own technique called "Instant Release," and the illumination method which is the blueprint for her own certification course "illumination."

She has an intuitive ability to lead people through guided meditations, visualizations, or conversations & communicate those messages that are exactly what they need to hear to clear physical, mental, emotional and spiritual blocks, reconnect deeper to their true self and higher power to shine their light brighter than ever before, and live their true purpose with more vision, confidence, and clarity.

She is passionate about assisting others in developing their gifts and reminding them that the answers are all within. "Be still, listen, meditate, then act. We are not alone; always remember your Angels and Higher power are all around to help you! Your success is Inevitable!"

 **SCAN QR CODE: Women's Health Class**

https://vimeo.com/806211101/885f121a3a

"Embrace Authenticity,
and Truly Live Your Essence."

Chapter 19:

Doing More by Doing Less

By Michael Vanderplas

T he constant hustle of the rat race is ever present in our daily lives. We have deadlines to hit, success to achieve. How the heck do I keep up with the neighbors? The pressure to do more, to be more, to achieve more is crushing. The stressors of the modern world seem to be augmenting all the time leading to a drastic increase of all mental health issues. Anxiety is running ramped, depression is an epidemic, and suicide rates are higher than they've ever been.

So how can we decrease our emotional stress and increase our mental health?

What if I told you that there is a way to achieve more by doing less? Would that be something in your life? What about the life of your loved ones? Of course, it would be.

What if you could learn how to realize the difference between what you really want and what you only think you want? What would that do for you in your life?

Lessons From a Legend

In early October of 2013 I stood outside the Lorraine Motel in Memphis Tennessee to honor a man that I had long admired. Martin Luther King Jr. His "I have a dream" speech has rung in the ears, hearts, minds, and souls of many of us for many years now. However, there are other sayings of his that I like even more.

"If you can't fly, run."

"If you can't run, walk."

"If You can't walk, crawl."

"But by all means, keep moving."

The reason why a lot of people never seem to move from good to great is because they don't give good enough a long enough chance for it to work. So often we are told the enemy of great is good. I couldn't disagree more. Without good, great would never exist. To get good at something, you need to first lay down the foundation by accomplishing smaller goals. Whenever you impose a superman syndrome and try too hard too early in the process, you'll never get the base level behaviors to stick.

Have you ever gone to the gym after not going for months or years and exercised extremely hard and long the first day back? How do you feel the next day or two? You know how you feel. You feel sore all over. Well, that's trying to be great without first trying to be good or even just okay.

If you want to run a marathon, you might want to run a 5K first. Want to lose 50 lbs.? Maybe eat 3-5 meals a day instead of starving yourself and binge eating late at night. Want to write a book? Start by writing 1000 words a day. That's what most great writers do. They don't worry about how good it is, they just write and know that a lot of it will be thrown away. You have the strength within you to do hard things. Just know that those hard things are so much easier when we do the easy things first. Realize that hard things usually are probably not getting easier. They're still hard. The only difference is that you are getting better, stronger. more skilled.

Doing More by Doing Less

So how do we overcome this strange tendency to hustle at a break-neck pace all the time? Well, that's easy, adopt the 90% rule.

I had an amazing (and very expensive) coach years ago. During one conversation, he pointed out that the reason I wasn't obtaining my goals was because I was trying too hard. Stephen told me that the highest that he ever aims for is 90%. I was shocked because he always seemed to be kicking butt in life. This guy charged $2,000/hour, has a Washington Post best-selling book, the wife and kid of his dreams and two INCREDIBLE cabins.

The more I thought about and adopted the 90% rule the more it made sense. No matter how perfectly you try to do something there is still something called life. And sometimes, life punches you right in the face and knocks you on your butt. This world is imperfect and therefore it is ridiculous to aim for perfection. Aim for 90%. I'm not saying to not try. I am saying that when we achieve 90% of any goal we set, we have made progress.

But what if we are not even able to give 90%? Then give 50%. Heck, give 50% of 90%. That's like 45%. It's still better than what you were doing before. It's also probably much more than what others are doing too. When we achieve ANY success, we feel accomplished. It builds self-confidence. That self-confidence decreases stress, anxiety and depression and therefore decreases the negative thoughts we might have previously thought about ourselves. Thus, leading us to a healthier, joy-filled life.

Perfectionism and Imposter Syndrome

So often we get worried about perfectionism. We are so hard on ourselves to be perfect, especially on the first try. But guess what, that will NEVER happen. In fact, it's impossible to do something perfect on the first try. For us to be great, good, or even okay at something, it takes practice. Right? Practice makes progress, not perfection.

Our strange internal desire for perfection is what prevents many of us from practicing the very thing we want to become perfect at. That's crazy. To become perfect, we need to practice, yet we don't want to practice because we are not perfect. It doesn't make any sense.

Those that become great are the same ones that were willing to aim for only 90% over a long period of time. Get out of your own head. You are not in competition with anyone else but yourself! Aim for 50% today and aim for 51% tomorrow. You are the only measurement of your own progression.

Too often we unknowingly get influenced by other people without even realizing it.

A few months ago, I got back from an amazing trip to Rome with my family filled with the best times and the best pasta of our lives. Upon returning home I tried connecting with five people that had professed their extreme excitement of "collaborating" with me in 2023. Two of them responded. The other three had vanished like Casper the friendly ghost.

At first, I was frustrated. I thought that they were going to be the contacts to push me over the precipice on my quest for millionaire status. A few days later, I realized that my life is freaking amazing and that maybe I don't need a million dollars. I realized that even though I didn't make a million dollars last year, I made enough to put me in the top 5% in annual income. In addition, I spend A LOT of quality time with my family. This changed me. I now know that I don't need to run at one hundred percent all the time.

A 2018 global study published by Perdue University looked at how much money appears to provide emotional well-being defined as the ability to control one's day-to-day emotional swings such as happiness, excitement, sadness, anger, fear, hurt and guilt. The study also measured life satisfaction. Worldwide, the study found that the ideal income for life-satisfaction is $95,000. For emotional well-being it's between $60,000 - $75,000. They found that any increase in annual income above that has very little impact.

Since I make well above that, I came to a life changing conclusion. I had been adding so much unneeded stress into my life because I felt that I needed to reach the same lofty goals as some of my friends and make one million a year. I had been stressing out seeing them reach their success and me not reaching their success. Some of them are making millions a year. Some of them are speaking in front of large crowds of people. Some of their sex lives are crazy and I wanted my life to be like theirs.

I was setting my goal at one million. But when I took a step back and took an inventory of my own life, I realized that I had what I really wanted. Sufficient money for my needs and wants. A loving wife and daughter. A meaningful career where I've helped save the lives of thousands both physically and emotionally.

I say this about me because I'm saying it about you. When you take an honest inventory of what your true, unconscious desires are and align your unconscious mind with your conscious mind, success (no matter how you define it) simply flows to you. When this happens, when the peace of mind arrives from you becoming your true authentic self and following YOUR purpose, your mental, emotional, physical and spiritual health all comes into balance.

Much Love and Stay Strong.

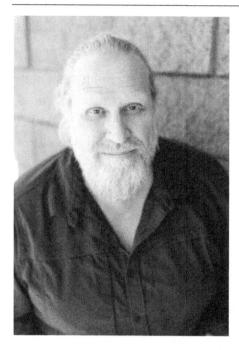

About the Author:
Michael Vanderplas

Michael Vanderplas Is a complete healer. As an ICU and Psychiatric Nurse for over 2 decades, Michael has been in more life-and-death situations than most. This has given him incredible insight into the total life spectrum.

Having flown over 1,000,000 miles, his coaching, public speaking, and trainings have taken him to Brazil, Guatemala, El Salvador, Mexico, Canada, Holland, and Australia.

In a lifelong quest to improve himself and those around him, he completed a long-time goal in 2017 to become a Certified Master Trainer of Hypnosis, NLP, and Quantum TimeLine Therapy.

In 2022 he became an International best-selling author with his debut book "Stay Strong - Overcome Suicidal Thoughts and Live the Life You Always Wanted."

Michael currently works on a daily basis with active-duty military service members, helping them overcome past and present traumas, build resilience, and form healthy relationships with others.

He provides life-changing breakthrough coaching sessions utilizing the most advanced unconscious mind mapping assessment tools on the market. He also provides training certifications in Hypnosis, NLP, and Quantum Timeline Therapy.

SCAN QR Code –

enlightened-academy.com/

YouTube: Viking nurse @vikingnurse4319

Instagram: mike_vanderplas

facebook.com/Michael.Vanderplas.NLP

"When You Become

the Master of Your Health,

You Become the Architect of Your Life."

Chapter 20:

The End

By Shelly Jo Spinden Wahlstrom

Done! *Now that your mind has been opened up to different options, you get to choose. It's not an either-or situation. There are so many different modalities to choose from. This book contains just a handful of experts. Now that you know this, you can continue on your journey to finding what works best for you.*

Mya Angelo stated, "When you know better, you do better." I encourage you to reach out to the experts in this book and learn more, get more information and work with those who resonate with you. Life is an amazing adventure. I've always believed that your body has the ability to heal when you find the right key for you.

Reminder: Life Matters…. You Matter!